Dear Liz and Wayne,
May this book brin[g]... of healthy cooking and eating together.
Wishing you all the health and happiness that you can handle,
Blessings,
Marie-Claire

Olives to Lychees
Everyday Mediter-asian Spa Cuisine
Volume 1

THE ART AND THE PLEASURE OF EATING WELL:
WHAT TO EAT, HOW TO EAT FOR OPTIMAL NOURISHMENT
AND WELLNESS TO RESOLVE HEALTH AND WEIGHT ISSUES

MARIE-CLAIRE BOURGEOIS

Copyright © 2015 Marie-Claire Bourgeois.

All rights reserved. No part of this book may be used or reproduced by any means, graphic, electronic, or mechanical, including photocopying, recording, taping or by any information storage retrieval system without the written permission of the publisher except in the case of brief quotations embodied in critical articles and reviews.

Please Note: This book is only intended to provide general information. It is not a guide for self-treatment or a substitute for medical advice, diagnosis or treatment by your physician or other health care professional.

The wellness suggestions and the recipes presented in this book are intended only as an informative resource guide to assist you in making the best informed decisions for you and your loved ones. For specific health concerns, medical questions, diagnosis or treatment, you should **always** consult your own physician and/or other competent health care professionals.

Please check labels carefully to confirm that the products you intend to use are in fact free of gluten and other "offensive" elements. Not all recipes in this book are appropriate for all people with celiac disease, gluten intolerance, food allergies or sensitivities.

Balboa Press books may be ordered through booksellers or by contacting:

Balboa Press
A Division of Hay House
1663 Liberty Drive
Bloomington, IN 47403
www.balboapress.com
1 (877) 407-4847

Because of the dynamic nature of the Internet, any web addresses or links contained in this book may have changed since publication and may no longer be valid. The views expressed in this work are solely those of the author and do not necessarily reflect the views of the publisher, and the publisher hereby disclaims any responsibility for them.

Any people depicted in stock imagery provided by Thinkstock are models,
and such images are being used for illustrative purposes only.
Certain stock imagery © Thinkstock.

ISBN: 978-1-4525-9923-6 (sc)
ISBN: 978-1-4525-9924-3 (e)

Library of Congress Control Number: 2014921160

Print information available on the last page.

Balboa Press rev. date: 2/19/2015

Table of Contents

Foreword i

Introduction ii

Part 1- The Problems: What Makes Us Ill and Gain Weight 1

Part 2- The Solutions: The Best Food to Eat Comes From the BASICS! 6

Part 3- The Art and the Pleasure of Eating Well 14

Part 4- Creating Your Own "EMaSC"--Your Everyday Mediter-asian Spa Cuisine to Nourish Mind, Body and Spirit During Your Spa Care Ritual and Every Day After 23

Starting the Day
Breakfast 24

While Waiting for the Next Meal
Snacks and Beverages 30

Whetting the Appetite
Appetizers 38

Warming the Soul
Soups 44

Loading Up on the Greens
Salads and Vegetable Dishes 51

Flying Protein
Chicken and Turkey 66

Grazing Protein
Beef and Lamb 71

Swimming Protein with Scales and Shells
Fish and Seafood 77

Satisfying the Sweet Tooth
1-Vibrant Fruit Desserts 82
2-Wholesome and Nourishing Baking 92

Gratitude 96

Resources and Recommended Reading 98

Index 99

Dedications

To all those who are struggling with health and weight issues,
despite their best effort to regain and maintain optimal wellness levels,
may this book offer a fresh mindset, answers and solutions.

To all those who don't know how to cook or don't cook much,
may this book offer the inspiration and the motivation
to develop this important life skill and have fun
preparing delicious and nourishing meals.

To all the health-conscious foodies who love to cook and eat fresh food,
may this book be a resource
for inspired creativity, optimal wellness,
and the Art and the Pleasure of eating well.

To Philip, my Sweet Love,
The best friend and most caring life partner I could ever wish for.
Thank you for always being so supportive in all my projects.
Feeling your loving presence next to me and hearing your steady encouragements
enable me to climb any mountain with confidence and perseverance.
I am at my best when I am with you.
You are my gentle giant.
Love you always.

M~C

Foreword

As *The New York Times Best-Selling Author* of many financial books over 30 years, I have made a career and a fortune teaching people how to be financially wealthy. I also teach my students that taking care of themselves is crucial to their financial success. As part of a healthy lifestyle, we all need to develop and practice a daily "rich-ual" consisting of physical exercises, nutritious meals, meditation, prayers, and positive affirmations to ensure that one's energy is grounded, positive, and receptive to divine guidance.

As I've often said, *Your Health is Your Wealth*. Anyone who has experienced illness would attest that without good health, it is more challenging to achieve your goals, and fulfill your life purpose. Investing in yourself and in your health is always encouraged as it ensures a brighter future. Along with a regular exercise program that suits you, one of the best health investments you can make is through proper nourishment and eating habits.

I met Marie-Claire at two of my "Fortune In You" workshops where she passionately introduced me to the concept of this book. She is absolutely amazing! Having the opportunity to try many different cuisines from around the world during my speaking and coaching engagements, I feel that this book is a timely gift to all of you foodies who love to cook and eat great food, and to those who want to learn how to cook real and fresh food to resolve health issues, and enjoy greater wellness.

In this book, Marie-Claire provides the reasons why, more than ever, we all need to nourish ourselves, as our ancestors did, with fresh produce from Mother Nature filled with antioxidants and life force energy, organically grown meats, the best oils, nuts and seeds. She guides the readers on how to take better care of themselves by adopting an improved nourishment-for-wellness plan, getting back to basics, and developing "the Art and the Pleasure of Eating Well", spa-style. She believes that a healthy lifestyle is the stepping stone to becoming more of what we are meant to be. Her creative ways of blending the amazing flavours of the Mediterranean and Asian regions into simple and healing dishes make this cuisine unique, timely and, best of all, healthfully delicious. The "clean" recipes will impress you and the people you cook for. You will feel well nourished and even pampered. It will transform your health and, ultimately, your life.

Robert G. Allen
#1 Best-selling author, speaker, mentor
The Fortune In You
Author of *Cash in a Flash*
www.RobertAllen.com
San Diego, 2014

Introduction

**Have you ever wondered why so many people
in North America, and more and more around the world,
are experiencing health and weight issues?
Perhaps, for our wellness, longevity and happiness,
we need to adopt a <u>fresher</u> approach
toward food, nutrition, and the Art and the Pleasure of eating well.**

*"We don't catch diseases;
we create them by breaking the natural defenses, especially the immune system,
according to the way we eat, drink, think and live."*
--Hering's Law of Cure

Why do women (and more and more men and children) go to the spa or the wellness centre? There are many reasons: a temporary escape in a peaceful atmosphere, a chance to de-stress and recharge, a few therapeutic treatments for health issues, a wellness class, a pampering treat, a special outing with a close friend or a loved-one, a delicious spa meal, etc. For some people, I wonder what excites them the most: going shopping or going to the spa?

For a long time, going to the spa was viewed as an expensive treat or frill that, if you were lucky, you would get to experience at least once in your life. We now know of the benefits a visit to the spa can provide, and, in a fast-pace lifestyle, these visits should be prescribed as part of a stress management and wellness program. The benefits I receive from my visits at the spa or at a wellness centre range from total relaxation and rejuvenation to an opportunity to do introspection, cleansing, and healing on many levels. I usually go back home with clarity of thoughts, a surge of grounded energy, a greater appreciation for my life, and new project ideas that I can't wait to explore. I feel high on life! I attribute these benefits to the sessions I received from the skilled therapists *and* the delicious and healthful spa food I ate. Eating delicious food is one of the greatest pleasures of life and, when it is combined with a sensual therapeutic massage (or other modalities) that makes you feel younger and vibrant, you reach a higher level of bliss and wellness.

With some planning and basic supplies, you can enjoy a "home spa" environment for regular stress release and pampering. For the day-to-day nourishing spa meals, this is where this book comes into play.

I am thrilled and honored that you chose to read my "nourishment-for-wellness" book. My intention is to share with you valuable information that could transform the aspects of your life that you feel need attention: your health, your eating habits, your weight, your energy level, and your stress level.

As a registered holistic health practitioner and a "nourishment foodie", I created this book for *you* to share delicious, nourishing and health-building recipes. I hope they will be valuable and life-changing for you and your loved ones so you can resolve some of your concerns (if not all of them), and remain healthy and happy.

When I think of *spa food*, I think of *less is more,* and I see:

- colourful and fresh food from Mother Nature, prepared simply and mindfully;
- visually attractive food that offers an enjoyable treat for the taste buds;
- high-energy food that has healing properties, and that provides essential nourishment and timely cleansing;
- controlled, mouth-watering portions that make me feel energized and satisfied as opposed to lethargic and stuffed.

By creating your own *"cleaner"*, *health-giving* and *nourishing dishes* at home, it is possible to enjoy *"comfort spa food"* (no, it is not an oxymoron!) every day -- or as often as you can -- *without sacrificing taste and pleasure!* I am inviting you to experiment with my collection of tasty nourishing recipes showcasing fresh produce and exciting flavours from the Mediterranean and Asian regions.

In this Volume, I will show you:

1. WHY it is important, *more than ever*,

   - to learn how to cook, if your skills are "under-developed";
   - to plan to cook your meals from scratch more often, using basic ingredients as nourishment powerhouses;
   - to know what to eat and how to eat by adopting a "fresher" approach towards food, nutrition and nourishment with my Paleo Nourishment and Lifestyle Plan to resolve and even prevent health issues; and

2. HOW you can make your Healthy Mediter-asian Spa Cuisine a part of your lifestyle to experience the Art and the Pleasure of Eating Well.

In **Volume 2**, I will focus on the Art of Feeling Well to deal with life's stressful challenges. You will learn:

- WHY creating a spa experience at home is important for your relaxation, stress management and wellness;
- HOW to nourish and rejuvenate mind, body and spirit by balancing your elements;
- HOW to develop your own Spa Care Ritual to get things moving when you feel *S.T.U.C.K.* using a few simple techniques and recipes to craft your own Mediterranean and Asian-inspired body care products;
- HOW easy it is to create your own Spa Cuisine to keep you hydrated and well-nourished; and
- HOW your Spa Cuisine can support your healthy lifestyle and the Art of Feeling Well during your pampering ritual and every day after.

Are your intrigued?
Is this what you have been looking for to remedy some of your health and weight concerns?
Can you envision a new wellness-based lifestyle for you and your family?
Can you imagine putting on the table colourful, fresh, aromatic and mouth-watering dishes that you, your family and your friends will love?
Can you see yourself creating these appetizing and healthy dishes with ease and comfort?
Can you visualize your life and your health changing for the better?
Take a moment to imagine what you want.

I bet you feel that you have been unwell, in pain and/or overweight long enough. Perhaps, being uncomfortable in your body has forced you to limit your activities, even put your life on hold. You have been looking for answers and solutions for quite some time. You have tried various diets and weight loss products without the lasting success you were hoping for.

We are all entitled to the healthy body we were born with, and to be happy. Unfortunately, the so-called modern Western diet and our eating habits are making us overeat, overweight, ill, and unhappy. They are reducing our longevity. It seems that the more we worry about nutrition – low fat, low carb, weighing food, counting calories -- the less nourished and healthy we seem to become.

Changing our eating habits and behaviour around food can be quite scary and stressful as they are so closely linked to who we are, our memories, our culture and our ethnicity. When we are forced to make changes, we want something quick and easy, like a magic pill or a formula, so we can go back to our regular routine, "magically transformed". However, as you know, science has not yet found a pill that promotes safe, healthy and lasting weight loss. Many people do not realize that there are no quick fixes to weight reduction and health recovery. Regaining health, maintaining it at an optimum level and preventing illness are part of a *process* and a *lifestyle* consisting of many little but meaningful steps and wise choices that reflect loving self-care, and commitment to the process.

No two people are built exactly alike and we "reset" ourselves repeatedly over time. It is never too late to make positive lifestyle changes in our lives. I would like to share my personal experience and my research on what you can do to increase your wellness, longevity and happiness. I hope to inspire you and your family to find -- or enhance -- your own equilibrium and healthy living so you can become more of your perfect, healthy and happy self. Perhaps you are one of the few wise individuals who are already living a healthy cooking and eating lifestyle. Congratulations! You are an inspiring role model. I believe that the content of this book will provide you with the information and resources to share with the people in your life who you feel might need some "enlightenment".

I believe that, despite our family history and genetic heritage, it *is* possible to redefine longevity. We *can* control how we live our lives. We can do that by focusing on our overall health, by understanding what the body needs, and by making choices that provide us with steady energy while supporting our long-term wellness goals. I feel that, more than ever, it is essential to become aware of the potential effect of what we ingest – good and not so good such as food, beverages, thoughts, news, visual images from the media, etc. -- on a daily basis as everything is energy in various forms and gets absorbed in the body's cells. If we want to experience steady and long-lasting health, we must have a nourishment plan based on quality natural and wholesome foods. We also need to invest more effort and money in building and preserving our health -- rather than in treating disease. We need to believe that Mother Nature is our best source for nourishment, remedies and healing.

My mission

To passionately share wellness and nourishment tips as well as easy and delicious recipes to support a healthy, happy and vibrant lifestyle. I want you *to fall madly in love* with healthy cooking and eating because playing with real food is fun and empowering. Healthy cooking gives you *clean gourmet dishes* that taste so good, nourish your body and brain, and provide you with plenty of grounded, happy energy to do what you want and need to do!

"Believe nothing.
No matter where you read it, or who has said it, not even if I have said it,
unless it agrees with your own reason, and your common sense."
-Buddha

I am a home chef and a "nourishment foodie" who feels that wholesome high-energy plant foods and superfoods from Mother Nature are the tastiest, most nutritious and healthiest. They also contain numerous wonderful healing and therapeutic properties. Choosing to live on plant-based, nutrient-rich foods is the perfect, easiest and most logical way to maximize nourishment while minimizing calories. It allows you to:

- Enjoy great food as a source of life-sustaining energy;
- Feel nourished *and* satisfied because increased nourishment equals less hunger and cravings;
- Reduce and manage weight more easily and naturally as you will be cutting down on empty calories and doubling up on your nourishment; and, if gaining weight is your goal, the plant-based nourishment might help you achieve it;
- Improve your digestion and elimination;
- Feel calmer and happier because your thoughts are clearer and the quality of your sleep has improved;
- Build health to resolve *and* prevent many debilitating illnesses;
- Take care of yourself, not as a form of self-indulgence but self-preservation. Self-care is not a luxury; it is rather a necessity. It allows you to connect to your heart, your soul, your nature and your essence (please refer to **Volume 2** for more information);
- Increase your energy and maintain it at a grounded, focused and steady level so you can concentrate on the meaningful things you want to accomplish as part of your life purpose;
- Increase your longevity and quality of life;
- Raise your vibration or frequency to enhance your connection with the Divine;
- Live your most creative and productive life;
- Positively influence the new generations of children and young adults to cook for themselves healthy, natural plant-based foods.

"Believe you can and you're halfway there."
-Theodore Roosevelt

As a young child, I didn't like food. I remember the challenge my parents had to make me eat. At around age 15, I gradually became interested in various flavours, and curious about how to put a dish together. When I moved out on my own, I started buying cookbooks on the different cuisines and taking cooking classes.

Because of my interest in nutrition and gastronomy, I have been cooking from scratch all my adult life. I find that the food I prepare myself is so much tastier, healthier and more satisfying (not to mention cheaper!) than the life-less, pre-packaged, store-bought versions. The money I save on cooking our own meals allows my husband Philip and I to purchase, among other things, fancier and better quality gourmet ingredients, like wonderfully fragrant and exotic vanilla beans, brightly coloured saffron, premium cocoa, fancy olive oil and balsamic vinegar, macadamia nuts, fresh seafood, organic produce and meats, etc. With basic ingredients, and some creative inspiration from a dish I ate at a restaurant or a recipe I saw in a cookbook, a magazine or on a cooking show, and with my personal touch, I can compose a dish that I am excited about and that pleases husband, family and friends. By the way, I read that according to some studies, *looking* at food pictures in magazines and cookbooks and *imagining eating* the food, will make you *eat less*!

> *"A good cook is like a sorcerer who dispenses happiness."*
> -Elsa Schiaparelli
> (We all have the power to cook great food that can dispense lots of happiness.
> Let's make us and our loved ones happier!)
> -Marie-Claire B

Throughout the years, I have been experimenting with several nutrition plans. I have been an omnivore, a "flexitarian", a vegetarian, a vegan, a "primal-paleo" eater, and a combination of them. Various stages of my life led me to change my nutrition plan, often because I wanted to shed some excess weight accumulated by the lack of movement due to minor sports injuries. All of these plans had a common healthy thread that I care about: lots of fresh *plant food*!

I am not a nutritionist or dietician. However, I consider myself a "natur-ian" and a "nourishment foodie". (I created these words to express my keen interest in delicious culinary creations full of nutritional value from Nature.) I read cookbooks and cooking magazines like people read novels. I come from a familial environment where everyone is an enthusiastic eater and cooks great food from scratch. In the small town where I grew up, there were very little convenience foods; therefore, everything was bought fresh and whole, and cooked at home. I consider myself lucky for inheriting a passion for good food, and for having been exposed to the art and skill of cooking. I, too, love cooking and eating real food that tastes so good, that satisfies and nourishes me, and makes me feel great. I don't count calories and don't know the biochemical value, mineral and vitamin content of any food. If I need to know that, I can look it up or ask a nutritionist. I just know that I can't go wrong living on a plant-rich nourishment plan. *The proof?* I feel great, I sleep well (most nights!) and I have lots of energy.

I LOOOVE real and fresh food, especially produce! I love their vibrant rainbow colours, their juicy-crunchy textures, their shapes and smells, their freshness that oozes wholesome goodness. And their delicious flavours. They are the first ingredients I think about when I plan a meal.

Why I Like Cooking

- I need to express my creative passion and, because I enjoy playing with food, cooking is a great outlet for me.
- Cooking makes me happy and I love to make people happy with my food.
- For years, I have been having this everlasting love affair with plant foods (produce) and the amazing Mediter-asian flavours.
- I feel like an artisan who crafts edible creations with great visual appeal by combining flavourful ingredients and infusing them with my personal touch and essence.
- A new kitchen tool that fits nicely in my hand is like a fun toy I can play with.
- My kitchen is my sanctuary, my atelier, and sometimes my sweatshop, depending on what I am cooking! (The results are always worth the effort!)
- I like to remember the countries Philip and I visited and to recreate the dishes we enjoyed while traveling.

I feel that cooking is a lot more than following recipes and putting ingredients together. It is more an emotional and intuitive activity than an intellectual one. A dish doesn't have to be fancy or fussy to be delicious and life-sustaining. I see my cooking as the fusion of the love and passion in my heart and soul and the essence of the fresh, raw ingredients – the end result being an enjoyable and memorable experience that appeals to the senses, and affects the heart and the soul of the people I cook for.

Part I- The Problems: What Makes Us Ill and Gain Weight

Inexplicable Aches and Pains; What's Going On in My Body?

A few years ago, despite my home cooking and health-conscious, mostly vegetarian nutrition plan combined with daily exercises, I was experiencing inexplicable stiffness, muscles aches, and burning bone and joint pains that were increasing in number and intensity, along with limited energy. Nothing was life threatening; just very annoying and puzzling. I certainly didn't want to continue living like that as I felt that the pains were worsening and restricting my activities. Taking medications to suppress the symptoms was out of the question! I knew that my body's built-in intelligence was telling me something. I had not suffered any serious injuries so I wanted to find the root causes before the discomfort became more incapacitating. I suspected that the inflammation I was experiencing was most likely triggered by some food intolerances, lack of sleep and increased stress, all causing higher acidity level in my body. I knew that the solutions and the remedies would come from Nature and my body's innate ability to heal itself, provided that I gave it all the opportunities to do so. One day that I was barely able to move, I decided that I had had enough discomfort. I was ready to take serious action, detox, and rethink my nourishment plan. I set an intention to find guidance and assistance.

Some Answers

In search of a non-drug pain relief solution, I found a practitioner of an energy-balancing technique* that I had been curious to experience: Matrix Repatterning®. By treating structural imbalances at the cellular level, this technique allowed me to feel calmer and more comfortable in my body so I could focus on finding answers to modify my lifestyle. After having asked my angels and the Universe, "What is the meaning of these pains that are waking me up at night? What do I need to know? What else can I do about them?" I was led to some answers. I came across the book *Wheat Belly** by preventive cardiologist Dr. William Davis, and I read it. It made so much sense to me that I immediately removed all wheat and gluten from my nourishment plan, for the second time. I had done so fifteen years before when I was studying holistic nutrition but I was missing today's science and research, and, eventually reintroduced wheat in my life. Within a week following the gluten removal, all my aches and pains disappeared, and I even regained overall flexibility, the range of motion in my shoulder *and*, as experienced fifteen years before, I was starting to shed excess weight!

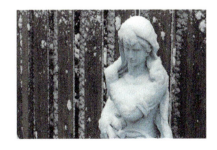

Dr. Davis asks, "Why has this seemingly benign plant that sustained generations of humans suddenly turned on us? It's not the same grain our ancestors ground into their daily bread. It has changed dramatically over the past fifty years under the influence of agriculture scientists. Wheat strains have been hybridized, crossbred, and modified so many times to make a wheat plant resistant to environmental conditions, such as drought, or pathogens, such as fungi. But most of all, genetic changes have been induced to increase yield per acre. The average yield on a modern North American farm is more than tenfold greater than farms of 100 years ago."

Because the wheat molecules have been genetically modified in laboratories over a thousand times, it is now a "frankenfood." These modified molecules act on the reward centre of our brain causing us to overeat even more and constantly crave more food; thereby, making us loyal consumers.

In *Wheat Belly*, Dr. Davis adds, "Wheat consumption has been linked to weight gain, especially belly fat, creating diabetes, inflammation, wheat addiction, and dozens of debilitating ailments. Wheat has infiltrated almost every aspect of our diet. One of the proteins in wheat, gliadins, crafted by geneticists, is an opiate**. Wheat is therefore an

---

* Please refer to the Resources and Recommended Reading section for the reference.
** According to *Merriam-Webster's Dictionary*, the definition of opiate is: "1) *a drug (as morphine or codeine) containing or derived from opium and tending to induce sleep and alleviate pain; 2) something that induces rest and inaction or quiets uneasiness.*"

opiate. Wheat keeps company with Oxycontin, heroin, and morphine. It has been known for a century that opiates, when administered to laboratory animals or to humans, increase appetite."

He also adds that if any form of inflammatory disease is present, such as rheumatoid arthritis or lupus, wheat is the gasoline on the fire, typically worsening inflammation and resulting in greater pain, swelling, skin rash, etc. Visceral fat is itself inflamed. If biopsied, it appears to be riddled with white blood cells, not unlike the pus that oozes from an inflamed wound. Visceral fat, or "love handles" or "muffin top", or "spare tire" also pours inflammatory proteins into the bloodstream, proteins that export inflammation out from visceral fat and into all other areas of the body.

"Wheat withdrawal closely resembles withdrawal from other opiates like morphine, Oxycontin, and heroin, just less severe. The effect generally lasts from 24 hours to several days, occasionally weeks," says Dr. Davis.

Contrary to the Canadian Food Guide suggesting that adults consume six to seven servings of grains per day, Dr. Davis recommends that we eat more fat and eat no "healthy grains", including wheat, to make diabetes recede.

Note: I have recommended the *Wheat Belly* book to at least a dozen people. Those who have read the book, avoided wheat and gluten as best they could, and found noticeable improvements in their pain and discomfort level. My neighbour Glenys was overjoyed when her doctor eliminated her recently prescribed diabetes medication! She was thrilled to report that she was also shedding some weight that, up until then, had been reluctant to melt. She is feeling transformed and very grateful! John, our residential handyman, also eliminated wheat and gluten from his nutrition and reported to me a few weeks later that he was feeling much fewer aches and pains and had been shedding some weight.

In the book *Fat Chance**, internationally renowned pediatric endocrinologist Dr. Robert Lustig documents the science and the politics that have led to personal misery and public crisis over the last thirty years: the pandemic of obesity and chronic disease.

In the late 1950's, when the U.S. government declared that we needed to get the fat out of our diets, the food industry responded by pumping in more sugar to make food more palatable and more salable, and by removing the fiber that makes us feel full, in order to make food last longer on the shelf. The result has been a perfect storm for our health, disastrously altering our biochemistry to make us think we are starving, drive our eating habits out of control, and turn us into couch potatoes. Dr. Lustig claims that if we cannot control how we eat, it is because of the catastrophic excess of sugar in our diet; and the resulting hormonal imbalances that have rewired our brains.

The more sugar we consume, the greater the craving for it, leading to increased levels of inflammation in our bodies. Like the nicotine in cigarettes, sugar is addictive as it activates the reward centres in the brain and produces dopamine.

In fat-free, low-fat or light versions of processed food, fat is replaced with sugar. These foods are often perceived as "guilt-free," causing people to overindulge. Dr. Lustig believes that the overindulgence in food and the high content of sugar in so many products are causing the pancreas, adrenals, and organs to be heavily taxed on a regular basis. Never in human history has there been such an assault on our blood sugar levels, resulting in many, if not most, diseases.

I heard on The Dr. Oz Show that "we now eat more than ever: on average between 2,200 and 3,000 calories per day." (That is a lot of calories when we know that 3,500 calories equals one pound.) Currently, "there are 1.5 billion obese people on the planet, which exceeds the number of starving people!"

In his book *Salt Sugar Fat**, Michael Moss, an investigative reporter, explains "how food scientists use cutting-edge technology in labs to calculate the *bliss point* of sugary beverages and to enhance the *mouthfeel* of fat by manipulating its chemical structure." He talks about the marketing campaigns designed from a technology adapted by tobacco companies to redirect concerns about health risks of their products: dial back on one ingredient, pump up the other two, and tout the new line as "fat-free" or "low-salt." He has talked to "concerned executives who confess that they could never produce truly healthy alternatives to their products even if serious regulation became a reality. He explains that the industry itself would *cease to exist* without salt, sugar, and fat. Just as millions of "heavy users," as the industry calls them, are addicted to this seductive trio, so too are the companies that peddle them. *No sugar, No salt, No sales!*"

Time to Cleanse

After eliminating wheat, sugar and processed foods (all acidifying foods) from your diet, you may still feel that some excess weight isn't coming off and some health issues remain. You might want to do some cleansing and look at other food intolerances to heal your digestive system, as it is crucial for optimal health. You might want to follow the program in *The Virgin Diet** book by nutrition and fitness expert JJ Virgin to eliminate the seven so-called "healthy" foods for three to four weeks (gluten; soy and corn -- both are GMOs; peanuts, eggs, dairy, and sugar). Reintroduce

---

* Please refer to the Resources and Recommended Reading section for the reference.

one item for one week, test (ingest), and notice. If the item is tolerated, it may be fine to consume on a regular or occasional basis. If not, *refrain* from eating it, as it may further damage your digestive system and bring back your symptoms and health issues. Then, reintroduce the next item. This book has been very helpful to me. After removing dairy, I noticed that I had more energy than ever before, and I was shedding extra weight that was, up until then, reluctant to melt despite regular exercise.

Since most of us have so many emotions related to food and eating, I invite you to take some time to ask yourself the following questions regarding food, eating, over-eating and weight issues. You may want to write down your answers in a journal. Keep asking the questions until you have uncovered all the answers inside of you. No judgment; just the truth. Once you have connected with the truth, you can make different choices to reach your wellness goals and, if necessary, ask for help.

- Why are you overweight? Why are you unwell?
- What is not working in your life?
- What makes you overeat? What are you hungry for? What kind of nourishment do you really need?
- Why do you want to lose weight and be healthier?
- Do you feel that you deserve to shed weight and be healthy?
- Do you have a support system?
- What would be the cost (physical, mental, emotional, spiritual, social, professional, financial) to you and your family if you did not lose the excess weight and regain your health?

More Answers

A few years ago, I experimented with a nutrition concept that has been gaining a lot of attention and traction: the Paleo Diet. The Paleo Diet* (short for Paleolithic, the earlier part of the Stone Age) is the first diet and lifestyle that the early humans survived on for thousands of years. It is based on the concept of eating the foods that were available from hunting and gathering: animal proteins (lean meats, poultry and fish), fruits and vegetables, nuts and seeds, before agricultural developments were made to grow grains and raise dairy cattle. It is believed that this ancestral way of eating -- *real, wholesome, nutrient-dense plant-food, as well as grass-fed and pastured meat* -- is what our bodies are designed to eat because it provides better fuel for more efficient and long-lasting energy, and therefore, burn fat. (A possible reason why this ancestral grain-free nutrition plan works could be that our genes have not adapted to cope with cultivated crops of modern agriculture.)

A lot of scientific research has been conducted by several leading experts on the benefits of adopting this nutritional framework to build stronger and healthier bodies. Just search the Internet; I leave the scientific explanations to the experts. This Paleo framework can be used as a template or guide to create your own nutritional plan with the foods that work best for your unique body and according to your tastes and preferences, so you can reach your personal wellness goals. The Gluten-free Diet alone didn't work for me because there are too many starchy carbohydrates and grains that replace the wheat in baked goods. I was concerned that, by eliminating the gluten intolerance problem, I would create another one: diabetes and serious weight gain as my body tends to hoard extra padding when I eat carbs and grains. It made the Paleo Nourishment and Lifestyle Plan perfect for me. Perhaps it will be perfect for you, too. It is worth a try.

As soon as I started following it, I began to feel satiated rather than stuffed and bloated after most meals. Within two weeks, my carb cravings were rapidly decreasing. And my digestive concerns, hot flashes, PMS discomfort, brain fog, migraine headaches, and the feeling of being mildly depressed and unhappy were fading away. The most significant improvement came when the aches and pains in my joints and bones, as well as the overall lack of energy,

---

* **What I think about the word** *"diet"*.

Words carry and emanate energy; just think of or picture the expressions "I LOVE YOU!" and "I HATE YOU!" Only the middle words are different. Notice what you think and feel.

"Diet" has the word *"die"* built in it; the French equivalent *"régime alimentaire"* (not much better) evokes restriction and rigidity. Both terms feel restricting, unpleasant, and *a temporary, unsustainable measure vs.* a permanent lifestyle improvement. I have not yet met a happy dieter. They usually look forward to the end of their diet to celebrate with some food they sorely missed. Some would say "I've been dieting for a month and all I've lost is a month!"

I prefer to use the term *"nourishment plan"*, referring to a more positive, uplifting and flexible approach that focuses, in a more relaxed way, on the enjoyment of abundant, tasty, healthy and satisfying food for a lifetime of nourishment leading to optimal wellness. So, I will refer to the Paleo Diet as the **Paleo Nourishment and Lifestyle Plan**, or the PNLP for short.

disappeared! I knew, then, that I had CRACKED THE CODE! I had found the answers I was looking for! Thank you, Universe! I now feel like the person I am supposed to be: happy and "high on life;" vibrantly healthy (confirmed by my naturopathic doctor); bursting with grounded, steady and focused energy; full of life and dreams. *Life is wonderful*!

Perhaps the answers I found to resolve my health concerns will be life transforming for you, too. Please continue reading to find out!

The Paleo Nourishment and Lifestyle Plan (PNLP) and Why I Feel This Is *Spa Food*.

The PNLP invites you to enjoy a variety of:

- pasture-raised and grass-fed meats;
- free-range poultry (preferably local or organic);
- game meats;
- pasture-raised eggs;
- fresh wild-caught fish and seafood;
- lots of nutrient-dense, fresh natural plant foods such as vegetables, fruits, nuts, seeds;
- healthy fats, i.e., cold-pressed extra-virgin olive oil, coconut butter, coconut oil, organic ghee, organic butter, avocado oil, macadamia oil, sesame oil, flaxseed oil, etc.

The PNLP suggests that you avoid:

- grains,
- legumes,
- soy and corn,
- processed foods,
- refined sugar,
- alcohol, and
- starches.

Eating *dairy* is very much an individual choice. The *Primal eating style* regards it as an acceptable food, while *Paleo* suggests avoiding it. If you are experiencing issues like a skin condition, an autoimmune disease, excess weight or lactose intolerance, avoiding dairy may be a wise decision that could prove to be effective in resolving or diminishing some – if not all -- of your health issues. If you have none of the issues mentioned above, occasionally consuming organic, pastured, full fat dairy can be an inoffensive treat.

Personally, I have "tweaked" these suggestions to suit my tastes and preferences for Mediterranean and Asian cooking. I choose to enjoy *very occasionally* some grains (mainly rice), and cheese in small quantity, mostly when entertaining, because we live in a modern world and many of my friends and family members still want to enjoy these foods. I see these foods as occasional treats for me. After I have enjoyed them, I go back to my regular PNLP and spa care because I feel so much better when I follow them on a daily basis. I will elaborate on this a little later. In this book and in **Volume 2**, I have not included any recipes with grains; however, a few recipes contain optional cheese, yogurt or cream.

A current medical concern may motivate you to improve your lifestyle and nutrition plan. Or perhaps you need to reduce your weight and maintain it at a more ideal level. Or you just want to maximize your health and longevity potentials. *There is no need to wait to become ill or develop food intolerances to experiment with the PNLP and a spa care ritual.*

By *avoiding* or *significantly reducing* your consumption of gluten, grains, legumes, starches, refined sugar, dairy, as well as processed foods and fast foods (all acidifying foods) and replacing them with fresh produce, (fruits and vegetables -- alkalizing foods), good quality meats, fish and eggs, nuts and seeds, and healthy fats, you might discover that you feel so much more energetic, lighter and overall healthier.

To create a more alkaline dinner plate, imagine that you divide it with a Y: the left and right sides (65-70% of the plate) filled with produce raw and cooked, nuts and seeds; and the upper part (30-35%) is reserved for quality meat, fish, eggs, and healthy fats. When your body is happy with its acid-alkaline balance, you might notice that you don't come down with colds or the flu anymore, or as often, because your immune system is getting stronger and is not as busy fighting the effects of offensive, highly inflammatory foods in your body. (For more information on how to measure your pH balance, and live a balanced-pH lifestyle, refer to the **Resources and Recommended Reading** section or surf the Internet.) Who knows what that extra energy and enhanced health will allow you to accomplish for you and your family, personally and professionally! I see the *PNLP* and a *daily spa care ritual* as excellent tools to achieve and maintain optimal wellness to live the life you want and deserve.

What Else Can The Proper Nourishment Provide You?
The Energy You Need to Live Your Unique Life Purpose.

"The purpose of your life is to find your gift.
The meaning of your life is to give it away."
- A Buddhist quote

Enjoying that extra energy and enhanced health could mean living your unique life purpose more fully, and having the courage to develop your unique gifts and to follow your most cherished dreams. It could also mean believing in yourself, being more positive and living with passion. In my opinion, a passion is ignited in the heart; it is both the fuel and the engine that make you feel alive with an enormous amount of uplifting, joyous and vibrant energy. A passion is what wakes you at night with inspiration, clarity and new creative ideas. It is something much bigger than you are; it has a life of its own.

"You have to discover you, what you do, and trust it."
-Barbra Streisand U.S. actress, singer

In order to stay vibrantly alive, you have to explore, nourish and experience that passion. If you don't, a part of you dies, un-actualized, disappointed, sad. When you explore that passion and let it grow, you feel alive, joyful and in the moment. Your spirits and your energy (or vibration) are high. You get totally immersed and absorbed in what you are doing, and time seems to fly by fast. Work doesn't feel like work; it is more like play. You don't think of checking the clock all the time. When you develop the passion in your heart, you start making a difference in the world around you. The changes in you will inspire the people in your life and encourage them to follow their own hearts. The positive and contagious influence you will have on others will trigger a chain reaction (or epidemic); and more dreams, joy and passions will be awakened which, in turn, will lead to more people being inspired to live their life purpose, and make a difference. And the contagion will spread, grow and become unstoppable (or incurable).

I believe that is how we can make the world a better place to live, learn and grow, just by starting this movement of becoming healthier and raising our vibration. The higher our vibration, the healthier we are. Also, we are all carriers of a uniquely bright light. It is up to us to dim it or allow it to shine and illuminate the world. Transforming the world into a brighter and better place starts with and within every one of us. This is the big picture that I keep in my mind when I share my passion for wellness and **optimal nourishment** *of body, mind and spirit, for a long, happy and vibrant life. For everyone.*

I invite you to visit my website www.mindyourbodyandspirit.com for a free copy of my Personal Transformation ebook *The REAL YOU: Your Gift to the World*.

"If we did all the things we are capable of, we would literally astound ourselves."
-Thomas A. Edison

Part 2- The Solutions: The Best Food to Eat Comes From the BASICS!

Why we need a "fresher" approach toward food, nutrition and wellness.

"Your food should be your medicine, and your medicine your food."
-- Hippocrates

"Overfed and undernourished", this is the result of following the modern Western diet. Without our consent or informing us, the government and food industries have made decisions that are greatly affecting our health and wellbeing. *We can get our power back by filling our plates with what WE want and need.*

Michael Pollan, a long-time contributor to *The New York Times*, and renowned author of several books on food, asks 3 questions:

What to eat?	*Eat food.* (I modify it a little: Eat "real" food.)
What kind of food?	*Mostly plants.*
How much?	*Not too much.*

Why Plant Foods Are So Important For Wellness and Longevity

I see plant foods and basic ingredients (nuts and seeds, honey, dark chocolate, eggs, sardines, etc.) as "power foods" or "nourishment powerhouses" because they are filled with the essential building blocks of nourishment. Numerous studies indicate that choosing to regularly eat vibrantly coloured fresh produce loaded with phytochemicals contributes to the prevention of major illnesses.

In his book *Eat to Live, the Amazing Nutrient-rich Program for Fast and Sustained Weight Loss**, Dr. Joel Fuhrman, a board-certified family physician specializing in preventing and reversing disease through nutritional and natural methods, recommends making vegetables (raw and cooked) the star, rather than the after-thought, to make the salad the main dish. Eat it first at lunch and dinner as you have a tendency to eat more of whatever you eat first because you are the hungriest. Raw food has more bulk, it will fill you up, and it has fewer calories. He also suggests to have at least 4 fruits every day (≈250 calories) for dessert or breakfast, to have one tablespoon of ground flaxseeds every day for omega-3 fats, and to consume about one ounce of nuts and seeds every day (≈200 calories).

Summer and early fall are the best times of the year to enjoy the abundance and the variety of fresh, seasonal produce that is full of *prana* (life force energy). It feels like a privilege to cook and eat vegetables, because they look and taste so good. There are so many great cookbooks and magazines to browse for inspiration, and delicious recipes to experiment with.

Dr. Fuhrman adds that the diet of most North Americans is only 5-6% nutrient-dense foods. Any step taken in the right direction will lessen the risks to their health. He believes that if the typical North American improves his/her diet now and begins consuming even 60% of his/her calories from nutrient-dense plant food – that is ten times as much vegetation as the average American consumes now -- it is reasonable to expect a 60% decrease in his/her risk of cancer and heart attack.

Once processed in the body, food has either an acidifying or alkalizing effect in the body, creating a change in the pH on the tissues and fluids. The term "pH" refers to the "potential for hydrogen." It indicates the concentration of hydrogen ions in a solution (i.e., saliva, urine, the blood affecting all cells in the body) measured on a scale from 0 to 14, 0 to 6 being acidic, 7 being neutral, and 8 to 14 being alkaline. To maintain optimum health, the body must be in an acid-alkaline balance. An excess of either bases can be fatal. Most people, because of their over-acidifying plant-poor eating habits, fast-paced and highly-stressful lifestyle, excess exercising or inactivity, have an overly acidic body that invites dysfunction and illnesses. With a diet that is mostly acidic, the body attempts to redress the imbalance by drawing on, and possibly depleting, its vital reserves of alkalizing minerals, -- calcium and magnesium -- from

---
* Please refer to the Resources and Recommended Reading section for the reference.

the bones and teeth. A nourishment plan based on plant foods would keep the body's pH in an ideal range; it would support the healing process, and enhance overall wellbeing.

In his *Nine Simple Steps to Prime-Time Health* DVD, Dr. William Sears explains that aging is like rusting because our bodies are oxygen-burning machines. Every minute, countless biochemical reactions throughout the body generate thousands of particles of exhaust called oxidants or free radicals that hit our tissues trillions of times a day like a steady rainfall, rusting away our cells.

He adds that this rusting of our cells contributes to chronic diseases like cancer but is also responsible for conditions associated with aging -- the ailments that many seniors complain about: hardening of the arteries, stiff joints, blurry vision, and wrinkled skin. Normally our bodies handle these free radicals by producing antioxidants or antirust chemicals, but when the body builds more oxidants than antioxidants, the rust accumulates and increases the wear and tear on the tissues. Unfortunately, as we age, our bodies tend to produce fewer antioxidants. Therefore, as we get older, we need to eat more foods that are rich in antioxidants; that means even more fruits and vegetables, and in a wide variety of them and of different colours.

He says that oxidation (rust), inflammation (wear and tear) and glycation (stiff and sticky excess sugar molecules that attach themselves to proteins and accumulate in tissues) contribute to many conditions of prime time: hardening of arteries, and all the "itises": arthritis, bronchitis, dermatitis, and "cognitivitis" -- Alzheimer's.

More reasons, I believe, to regularly consume much more plant foods that are packed with antioxidants, essential nutrients and life energy to slow down, delay and even stop the development of diseases in our bodies.

Why Mother Nature Made the Produce So Brightly Coloured

There are five bright colour groups of produce and each one is associated with one or more phytonutrients. Did you know that the brighter the colour, the richer the food in nutrients? Each colour of the rainbow spectrum releases or emanates a different energetic vibration. Our organs, glands and chakras (energy centres) respond to these vibrations. When we eat large amounts of fresh and colourful produce, we have a greater chance of absorbing sufficient life force that has a high energetic vibration. As I mentioned earlier, the higher our vibration, the healthier we are. The fresh and colourful produce help us cope with our stresses and thrive, allowing us to continue living at a high energy level. I think that their 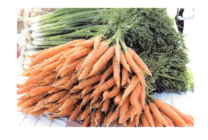 attractive bright colours are meant to catch our attention and to remind us that we need to eat them daily! Aim to make your plate colourful at every meal.

- **Red** Some red foods (like tomatoes, watermelons, pink guavas, red grapefruits, red papayas) get their colour from lycopene, which may reduce the risk of lung, stomach, and prostate cancers.
- **Yellow/orange** These colours tend to indicate the presence of beta-carotene, which may help prevent heart disease as well as lung and colon cancers. Produce displaying these shades are carrots, apricots, cantaloupes, mangoes, papayas, peaches, persimmons, winter squashes, sweet potatoes.
- **Green** Fruits and vegetables in this colour, especially the dark green ones, often contain several phytonutrients like the eye-protecting lutein, and beta-carotene. Produce in that colour group include collard greens, kale, bok choi, broccoli, cucumbers, Swiss chard, peas, romaine lettuce, spinach, zucchini, kiwis, green grapes.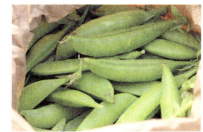
- **Blue/purple** Foods in these hues are rich in anthocyanins, and phytonutrients. Foods like blackberries, black currents, figs, apricots, blueberries, plums, red cabbages, beans, carrots, red onions have anti-aging and anticancer properties, and assist the circulatory function.
- **White** Foods like garlic, leeks, onions, and shallots are part of the allium family and they contain allicin which boosts the immune system. Some contain quercetin, a natural anti-inflammatory agent.

My Spa Cooking Style

It consists of 5 must-haves: ***quality and freshness, variety, quantity, visual appeal,*** and ***olfactory and gustatory appeal.***

Creating delicious dishes with fresh produce that will keep your taste buds interested and delighted is not complicated or challenging. You don't have to be a seasoned chef to cook great food that everyone will love. In fact, cooking real food is very simple, satisfying and so tasty. It is the ***quality*** and the ***freshness*** of the ingredients that will make a dish outstanding and spa-like – ingredients that are the freshest and the most beautifully coloured. Food that is good for us is the simplest in its "naked" form, *"au naturel."* Just adding a pinch of grey Celtic salt (or you can use as a finishing touch *sel de Guérande* -- non-refined salt full of minerals from the sea, hand-collected according to an ancestral French method, -- or *Fleur de sel*, all available in most grocery stores), freshly ground black pepper, a handful of fresh herbs, pinches of spices, and a splash of extra-virgin olive oil, flaxseed oil or lemon juice, is all that is necessary to enjoy the full flavour of fresh vegetables. You can also choose a simple cooking method, such as steaming, broiling, grilling, poaching, roasting, braising, stir-frying, or leaving the vegetables in their raw nature, which means less work in the kitchen. To accompany and enhance the vegetable dish(es), I like to add a small amount of protein, the size of my palm, more or less, a few handfuls of nuts and seeds, herbs and spices for added satisfying low-calorie flavours and antioxidants. Very often a snack or a dessert is as simple and natural as a fresh ripe fruit.

Every season brings us its fragrant and flavourful delicacies from Mother Nature, either grown locally or on foreign lands. So there is a lot to choose from year-round, and the combinations are endless. Furthermore, choosing to live on a nourishment plan based on an abundance and ***variety*** of fresh, ripe fruits and vegetables will provide most of the fiber, minerals and vitamins, phytonutrients and antioxidants, proteins and carbohydrates, as well as the acid-alkaline balance that your body requires. My cooking varies according to the seasonal ingredients. For instance, when it is peach season, I find ways to incorporate the juicy, fuzzy treat into breakfasts, salads, salsas, meat dishes and, of course, desserts. Moderation and portion control allow us to enjoy all foods in small amounts without serious consequences. I often opt for the *"less is more"* approach to determine the ***quantity*** I want and need to consume. Since the ingredients I choose are super fresh and tasty, a small amount of the prepared dish is sufficient to satisfy my taste buds and my appetite. We can all function well and be healthier with a little less food.

We eat with our eyes first, so the dish must have very colourful ***visual appeal.*** The presentation must show loving care, otherwise it can look like a steaming mess fit for a dog's breakfast.

When I start playing with food, my five senses spring into action; I see cooking as quite an experiential, organic and (even orgasmic) activity. I often get very excited about the various textures in my hands as I prepare the raw ingredients, the beautiful colours of the vegetables becoming more vibrant as they cook, the intoxicating aromas (*olfactory appeal*) that emanate from the juices being released when meat and vegetables are being cooked or when various ingredients marry together, the unmistakable sounds announcing chemical transformations of the ingredients as they heat up. And when the finished product comes in contact with my taste buds (*gustatory appeal*) and explode in the desired tastes and textures…Ooooh!... What an orgasmic reward for my effort!

Instinctively or intuitively, I gravitate to produce -- or plant-food as I like to call them – for the life force energy or *prana* and the antioxidants they provide the body. The more vibrantly coloured they are, the more antioxidants they contain. They form the best preventive medicine.

Other Forms of Nourishment for Optimal Wellness, Longevity and Happiness

In this holistic or wholistic (meaning *whole vs.* separate and individual parts) nourishment book based on real and fresh food, I could not omit to mention other aspects of body-mind-spirit nourishment that contribute to adding years to our lives and vitality to our years, while enhancing the quality and enjoyment of our day-to-day living. The secret is to find and maintain regular habits that make our bodies happy, and that we can sustain throughout life for optimal wellness and longevity. These habits become part of a healthy lifestyle that we can enjoy and thrive on because they help us manage and balance our energies. Following are a few of many possible healthy habits. See which ones currently feature in your lifestyle, and which ones you feel, if you added them, would make a positive difference in your wellness and happiness.

A) Physical Activity and Movement

Our bodies are designed to move. They need the right type of movement in the right quantity and frequency. They serve us much better when we give them adequate and regular movement, by *being active and in motion throughout the day*, in the form of an exercise, a sport or an activity, especially one that we *moderately* to *truly* enjoy. If your job requires you to sit most of the day, it is important to frequently get up, stand, stretch and move as much as possible to increase your energy level and blood circulation, especially in your legs.

A regular program of exercise combined with an improved nourishment plan contributes to increase fitness and maintain overall wellness. The benefits of regular physical activity are numerous and well known now. As you probably know, regular exercise helps to:

- burn calories more efficiently, and take off excess pounds,
- replace fat with muscles, and give your body a firmer and more youthful look,
- increase your cardiovascular system,
- increase the blood flow to your brain,
- improve the mood,
- release stress and tension, to relax and calm the mind,
- increase your metabolism and overall energy,
- reduce your appetite,
- regulate your blood sugar.
- And, as you get hot and sweaty, you feel high on life because of the endorphins -- the feel-good hormones -- that are released while you huff and puff!

Many studies have shown that even walking at moderate speed for 20-30 minutes daily can increase our longevity by three years as it potentially reduces the risks of cancer (i.e., colon, breast, and lung) and cardiovascular diseases. Performing regular movement or exercise ensures better quality of life and autonomy as we age. It can delay and even prevent years of invalidity when simple activities like taking a shower, getting dressed and running errands become challenging. Among the body changes associated with aging, bone mass and muscle mass losses, osteoporosis, and heart disease can be prevented or delayed with regular physical activity and movement throughout the day. It is believed that regular physical exercise and movement promote the oxygenation and the improvement of our brain functions that help us preserve our cognitive vitality and memory. It is never too late to start being active; your whole body will benefit.

"The slower we move, the faster we die. Make no mistakes, moving is living."
-George Clooney, as Ryan Bingham in the movie "Up in the Air" (2009)

My body tells me very clearly when I haven't moved enough. While working on these books, many times in very clear ways, my body expressed its unhappiness at the lack of sufficient and adequate movement. Therefore, I have to remind myself to get up and move around because I know that the longer I sit, the less energetic I feel, mentally and physically. Most days, I do some movement preferably outdoors in the sun to uplift my spirit and to maintain adequate vitamin D level. Moving to fast-paced music energizes me; I get to raise my heart rate, sweat and activate muscles, joints, and spine. I love to dance and, for fitness, I developed my own unique intense style in the privacy of my home: trashing around, disturbing the dust and fogging up the window! It is not very pretty, but it is effective and exhilarating. You should try it! Or have some kids show you how. Keep in mind that *a kid* can be a 75-year young person. Be a kid again and shake it up! It does magic for the spirit. Please refer to **Volume 2** about Soul Dancing and other ideas to move the body.

Have you danced lately?

I also enjoy doing interval training on the rebounder (or trampoline) with upbeat music playing loud enough so I can "feel" it. I find it to be a short workout that is easy and quite effective. Here is what I do: for this interval training, I warm up by jumping on the rebounder for 10-15 minutes. (If you don't have a rebounder, you can start with a warm-up of your choice and proceed with the interval training on the floor, or doing a walking-jogging combination.) Then, using a clock, I start a cycle of fast jogging on the rebounder for 20 seconds, followed by a "pause" of regular jumps for

10 seconds. Believe me; a cycle goes quite fast, especially the "pauses"! I aim to do 8-10 cycles which amounts to a total workout of 4-5 minutes. It doesn't sound like much; however, it makes you feel hot, sweaty and panting, but GREAT!

What is important is that you move your body with an activity that you love and you do it on a regular basis for the rest of your life, or until you find another type of movement that you are excited about and can sustain. And a couple of times a week, you lift heavy things for strength training. A good *physical movement program* should have a balance of strength and endurance, flexibility and agility, coordination, and rest periods. Also, in order to be able to move for life, it is important to respect your body and its physical limits, and to listen when enough is enough. Have a back-up plan if you are nurturing an injury and you want to remain active. Movement is essential to keep the body fluids flowing freely, and to help push toxins and bacteria out of the body. Yoga and a gentle walk, or any other low-impact activity that you can easily do and enjoy, could consist the basis of your movement program onto which you add other forms of exercise for strength, endurance and coordination.

Have you shaken your bootie today?

For my wellness, I use 5 key things: a *journal* to record my movement and plant food consumption, a *scale* for weekly weigh-in (so a 2-lb gain doesn't turn into 20 pounds), a *pedometer* to record my goal of at least 10,000 steps per day. And to ensure that things are moving and flowing smoothly, lots of *fiber*, and plenty of *water* (2-4 L per day). By measuring and recording, I have a greater chance of keeping up with my routines. My nourishment plan allows me to have steady, positive energy. Regular exercise helps me use that energy effectively and generate more.

B) Rest, Relaxation and Breathing

"All human evil comes from this: a man being unable to sit still in a room."
-Blaise Pascal

The right balance between exercise and rest helps to maintain our bodies in a more alkaline state. *Scheduling some time to have nothing scheduled* is necessary to maintain a proper balance between activity and *down-time*. We were not designed to go-go-go and experience prolonged stress. For optimal function, our bodies and mind-brains need daily inactive periods for the 5 Rs: Relaxation, Rest, Repair, Rejuvenation or Renewal of our energies, and Recreation or *Re-creation* – finding time to let go, disconnect, have fun and re-create ourselves. In **Volume 2**, I share suggestions on how to create a daily spa care ritual to ensure you get the well-deserved relaxation that you need to feel well.

"Stress is an ignorant state. It believes that everything is an emergency. Nothing is that important."
-Natalie Goldberg, author and writing instructor

If relaxing is difficult for you because you are worried about a situation, one way to move on from it, and put your mind at ease, is to acknowledge it by writing it down on a piece of paper. Write the possible solutions that you are considering. Then, take several deep breaths and ask your Inner-Wise Guide (we all have one) and the Universe or the Source or God to have other (or better) solutions revealed to you in some way that you will be able to recognize them as the solutions. Trust that the answers will come to you in due time. Then, since you did something about your worry (you brainstormed for solutions and asked for assistance), let it go and occupy your mind with something fun and distracting.

"Man is ill because he is never still."
-Paracelsus (Often quoted by Dr. Randolph Stone, founder of Polarity Therapy)

Here is how you can connect with stillness – a concept that can feel quite foreign to you if you have been on overdrive for most of your life -- and recharge your mind, body and spirit. This is a very easy and simple meditation that you can practice anytime, anywhere. For two minutes (and we can all find two minutes in the day), with your eyes closed, you do nothing but sit still and focus mindfully on your breathing: place a hand on your belly and feel it going out as you inhale, and feel it going in as you exhale. Observe the thoughts that cross your mind, acknowledge them and imagine them as passing clouds in the sky, coming and going. Then, bring your focus back to your belly breathing. This exercise trains your mind to focus on one thing: keeping your awareness on your breathing. Gradually increase the still time by adding one minute; then, two minutes, up to 20 minutes or more. Many different thoughts will cross your mind. Eventually, an idea or an answer that you were looking for will appear. Whenever you need to break away from the rat race of our modern lives, focusing on your breath while sitting still can help you slow down your pace and heart rate. If you would like to experience a relaxing guided meditation or learn about Polarity Therapy, visit my website at www.mindyourbodyandspirit.com or refer to **Volume 2**.

"Meditation is not an escape from life, but preparation for really being in life."
-Thich Nhat Hanh

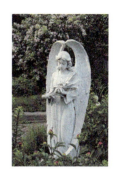

Your breath connects you with your body and the present moment. When you worry, you are in your head revisiting the past and/or imagining and anticipating stressful scenarios that have not taken place. We all do that when we are stressed or worried or hurt. Being aware of it and bringing our focus to the body and the present can drastically reduce the time spent in the stress mode. Here is an energizing way to start the day: while still in bed, for five minutes, focus on your breathing to energize your body and align your thoughts in a positive direction for the day – focusing on what you want. At mid-day, you can re-centre and ground yourself for five minutes. And finish the day, in bed, with 5-10 minutes of focused breathing before falling asleep. As you relax, feel gratitude for everything in your life – blessings, successes, lessons, challenges, gifts, etc. Imagine how you want the next day to be. You might notice that you are feeling more relaxed and grounded, your blood pressure is lowering, the tension in your body is easing, your mind is clearing, your thoughts are calmer and more positive, and your sleep is more peaceful and uninterrupted.

"The quieter you become, the more you can hear."
-Ram Dass

Taking the time to do focused breathing is like putting gas in the tank of the car. We cannot afford not to do it if we want to keep going. On extremely busy and stressful days, we need to do it twice as long! There are many wonderful things occurring during stillness: the body does its repair work, and our mind chatter diminishes to leave space for inspiration, insight, and guided actions coming from our Inner-Wise Guide. The effect of a few minutes of stillness on the body and the mind is equivalent to a couple of hours of restful sleep. What could be better?

"Within you, there is a stillness and a sanctuary to which you can retreat at any time and be yourself."
-Hermann Hesse

C) Sleep

Numerous studies have found links between poor *sleep* quality and difficulty shedding weight. Sufficient quality sleep helps to maintain healthy heart function, and to balance metabolism and hormone levels. It is crucial to have sufficient quality sleep most nights for a healthy weight, wellness, and… mood! Studies have shown that long-term sleep deficit increases the risks of depression, and even leads to obesity and diabetes. Good sleep allows our brain to rest. It protects our mental health, strengthens our memory and enhances what we learned during the day. (I know that when I don't sleep well or enough, I am not fun to be around the next day. I can't focus or think straight, and I have no patience. It negatively affects my food choices and my motivation to exercise.) In order to recover from and compensate for the nighttime sleep deficit, taking a nap during the day may be a wise solution. Going to bed earlier the following night is another one. Think of sleep as a form of nourishment for your body and your brain. Don't let yourself go hungry for sleep.

"The beginning of health is sleep."
--Irish proverb

D) Developing and Stimulating New Neuro-pathways

No doubt you have heard or read that, in order to preserve our brain health, it is essential to keep mentally and intellectually active and stimulated. Numerous studies have shown that nourishing our brain with activities and tasks that are stimulating reduces our risk of developing cognitive illnesses like Alzheimer's. In fact, remaining mentally active increases the number of neuro-networks and possibly the number of synapses in the brain, creating a cerebral reserve against mental illnesses. Activities like working at a stimulating job, enjoying an intellectually interesting pastime, taking courses to continue learning, performing memory exercises regularly, finding solutions to challenges or puzzles have all proved to be beneficial in keeping the brain active and sharp.

What are you doing to keep your brain active and healthy?

You may find that the more physically active you are, the more alert and smarter you become. Learning and remembering, among many benefits, are enhanced through physical movement. Over three decades ago, through extensive research in education, psychology, and neural and muscular function, Dr. Paul Dennison and his wife Gail created Brain Gym®: a movement-based educational experience centred around 26 simple activities that recall the movements children naturally do during their first years of life as they learn to coordinate their eyes, ears, hands, and whole body. Dr. Dennison says that *"Movement is the door to learning!"* Around the world, people of all ages use the learning program Brain Gym to bring about rapid and often dramatic improvements in their reading, writing, language, and numerical skills. Other people use the work to deeply enhance the quality of their attention and concentration, relationship and communication, memory and organizational skills, athletic performance, and more. For more information about Brain Gym, visit my website at www.mindyourbodyandspirit.com. To find Brain Gym classes or a consultant near you, visit www.braingym.org.

E) Social Circle

At any age, a strong social circle can help us maintain our mental health and keep us stimulated with intellectual activities like gatherings, discussions, outings, hobbies, etc. A supportive and energizing social network is essential for personal growth, enjoying life to the fullest, and as a comforting cushion to fall on during challenging times. Maintaining a strong social network helps us reduce our stress and anxiety levels; it lifts our spirits. We were not put on this earth to experience life on our own. We need one another for wellness, happiness and longevity. Life is more fun when we can share it with caring family members and supportive friends. Being with people that we care about and who make us feel great is nourishing to the soul and the spirit.

"A journey is best measured in friends rather than miles."
-Tim Cahill, U.S. author

F) Decluttering, Letting Go, Detoxifying

Regularly shifting, reorganizing and discarding our accumulated earthly things keeps the energy flowing freely in our environment. Anything broken or stained that can't be fixed or cleaned, clothes that don't fit well, and anything that doesn't bring you happiness and enjoyment can be donated, recycled or discarded. This purging makes room for new items to enjoy. Or you might decide that you prefer the space open and free. After *decluttering* and cleaning the house, the energy feels fresh, clearer, and free-flowing. It is especially beneficial in the spring and before New Year's Eve to make room for fresh energy to enter the home.

Re-evaluating our relationships by choosing those that are supporting and stimulating, and letting go of those that are negative and energy-draining can be one of the best things we can do to ensure that our energy levels and vibration remain high. The relationships that need to end -- or dissolve on their own as we stop investing energy in them -- are those we have with individuals who don't make us feel good, are never available when we need them, and do not appreciate what is important to us. *Letting go* of these relationships can be quite liberating and healing. The quality relationships to treasure and nurture are those with the people who inspire, motivate and uplift us, especially when we are not at our best. They accept and value us. They are grateful for what we have to offer. They bring out the best in us. When we spend time with them, we feel joy, respect and love. They bring value into our lives as we do in theirs. We can't get enough of each other!

"Strive to be first: first to nod, first to smile, first to compliment, first to forgive."
-Anonymous

It seems that more and more young people are experiencing health issues: joint pain, skin problems, mood disturbances, menstruation and fertility issues in women, allergies, susceptibility to infection, autoimmune disease, etc. *Detoxifying* the body by removing the unwanted waste products is important to maintain optimal health, longevity and happiness. Most people take better care of their cars with regular maintenance check-ups than they do of their bodies. Spring and fall are ideal periods of the year to detox the body but more frequent detox programs -- one day a week, one day a month, one week per season – can also be considered depending on your lifestyle, needs, and motivation. Good health comes from good digestion function and regular bowel movements (without relying on laxatives), detoxifying and rebuilding. In **Volume 2**, I share Dr. Stone's **Polarity Purifying Diet** that I personally use and recommend to my clients. It is a very gentle, easy to use and effective cleansing method to feel better and healthier. During and after a cleanse, you might notice that some of your health concerns are lessening and even disappearing. The key is to determine what works and adjust your lifestyle. Many health issues can be resolved by eliminating offensive and inflammatory foods. Planning regular cleansing spa days or spa weekends at home that include loving care "treatments," gentle exercises and health-building meals for you only or with a friend or your spouse can be therapeutic, and have the effect of a relaxing mini vacation. More and more men are now enjoying and appreciating pampering treatments.

G) Having Fun

A sense of humour certainly helps make life more enjoyable and the challenging times more bearable. Laughing engages many muscles (face, torso), lowers blood pressure, reduces the stress level, strengthens the immune system, and releases endorphins -- the feel-good hormones. A good laughing session can feel like a painless workout, and require an urgent trip to the bathroom! If you watch children play, you will notice that they laugh and giggle more frequently and whole-heartedly than adults. Somehow, as adults, while attempting to be more mature and taken seriously, we have neglected or lost the natural ability to be spontaneous, happy, and take ourselves and life more lightly. To compensate for this, finding a fun outlet can do wonders for the spirits, the overall mood, and stress levels. I think that a laughing face is the most beautiful sight: wide-open mouth revealing teeth and tongue, eyes looking like half-moons from which joyful tears often trickle down. The overall energy is engaging. It is pretty difficult to remain indifferent in front of a smiling or laughing face. Often, all we need is someone to start giggling and having fun, and a contagious laughter is spreading. Everyone wants to be part of it.

What do you do to have fun on a regular basis? Do you, like me, collect funny jokes that you read once in a while? Do you like watching comedy movies or shows? When was the last time you truly had fun? What did you do?

I think that children and pets are our best teachers and play buddies as they are in a perpetual state of *CRA – Cheerfully Ready and Available!* Their spontaneous nature reminds us of what it is like to have fun. They can inspire us to get back to this natural therapy of stress release and overall wellness. Laughter is the best medicine. Have you had your daily dose today?

> *"The doctor of the future will give no medication,*
> *but will interest his patients in the care of the human frame, diet, and in the cause and prevention of disease."*
> -Thomas Edison

Part 3 - The Art and the Pleasure of Eating Well

How we can make the "fresher" approach a part of our lifestyle

"To eat is a necessity, but to eat intelligently is an art."
- Duc de La Rochefoucauld, French writer

My Experience with the Mediter-asian Lifestyle

Both my mother and Philip's mother produce great meals on a daily basis in quite small kitchens. My mother's tiny U-shaped kitchen is so cramped that when two people are moving around, they inevitably bump *derrières*. Lily Ma's kitchen is more open but has practically no counter space or storage cupboards. Yet, their limited cooking spaces don't stop these amazing octogenarians from being comfortable enough to cook great meals every day. In fact, it is in their kitchens that you will likely find these ladies, most of the day. It is the gathering place of the house where you feel warmth, love and comfort, where you can always find a tasty treat, and where great conversations take place. Have you ever been to a house party and everyone converged in the kitchen because that was where the conversations were the liveliest and most engaging?

I cook something from scratch every day. When I am inspired, I cook even more. I get my inspiration from food pictures, cookbooks, cooking magazines, Philip (when he says "You haven't made this dish in a while…"), and a trip to the grocery store. It is when I started traveling to France, Italy and Spain that I realized the lifestyle of cooking and eating that I grew up with is similar to that of most European people: the love of great food, the pride in cooking it yourself to ensure the best flavour, the joy of sharing the resulting feast with family and friends as a celebration of gratitude to life and Mother Nature, and *la joie de vivre* (the enjoyment of life).

Like the European people and the Chinese people I know, I go grocery shopping a few times a week for fresh ingredients and inspiration to answer the quotidian question, "What's for dinner?" Often, I go to the supermarket for a few ingredients and come home with several more because of the new meal ideas that I "saw" in my mind while walking the periphery of the store. It takes just a little longer to put a fresh salad together, steam some vegetables while a few pieces of chicken are baking in the oven, than it takes to thaw and microwave a frozen dinner. And to round off this healthy repast, a dessert made with seasonal fruits is deliciously simple and quick.

While growing up, I was used to seeing friends and family come to visit my parents and stay for lunch or dinner; it seems that there was always enough food for one or two unexpected guests. To this day, neighbours walk over to my parents' house for a chat and end up sharing an impromptu meal with them, a phenomenon that I rarely see or hear about in the big city as people seem to be too busy with things to do, places to go and texts to read.

It is through my travels as an adult that I came to understand and appreciate my family's approach to great food and eating well. I realized that, like the Mediterranean folks, my parents and grandparents know the importance of making time to cook great food for family and friends, living well and sharing their abundance. They know that this type of lifestyle nourishes not only the bodies but the souls as well. They believe that speed should not be a priority because when you are enjoying yourself with great company and nourishing your body with lovingly prepared food, why would you want to rush cooking and eating? I found that this more healthful approach to food and living well is very much ingrained in their nature, their souls and their socio-cultural fiber, 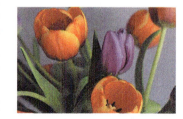 even though none of them ever set foot in Europe! I am very grateful for this rich heritage and the art of eating and living that they have passed down to me, and as a result, the health I have been enjoying.

I love planning a menu, and setting up the dining environment or the "stage for feasting, chatting and bonding" – dining room, garden, balcony, beach, picnic blanket, classroom, anywhere! From my mother, I inherited my love of setting a nice table that is inviting and attractive with tablecloth, *soft* cloth napkins (not the rough paper or synthetic ones that make you want to use your shirt sleeve instead), real dishes and cutlery, crystal glasses (it is amazing what you can find during clearance sales!), candles (for breakfast, too!), fresh flowers from the garden, music, and festive decorations to mark a special occasion. It elevates the dining experience to a level of celebration, greater enjoyment and appreciation. (I admit; any excuse is a good one to gather some people and celebrate with food!) I believe that since I spent time and energy preparing the feast, my creative efforts deserve to be lovingly presented and showcased on a pretty table. It doesn't take much longer to set the table and clear it after the meal. Most guests are more than happy to help, and family members are *trainable!* I am lucky, Philip is always helping. When I thank him, he responds, "Why not! I'm eating, too. Besides, it's faster with two people."

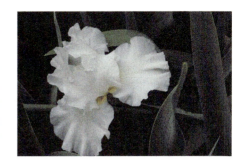

Strategies to Ease Into (or Enhance) the Art and the Pleasure of Eating Well

A) Shopping

- *Plan your meals and snacks* for a few days or the week. Make a shopping list of the ingredients needed and stick to it!
- The easiest and safest way to ensure that the foods with which you fill your refrigerator and pantry are free of "junk" (MSG, chemicals, colouring, excess salt and sugar), GMOs and wheat-grain-gluten, is to *focus on basic fresh and natural, single-ingredient foods*: produce from the grocery store or the fruit and vegetable stand at the farmers' market, or your garden, the meat from the butcher shop, the fish and seafood from the fish store.
- *The best food to eat is found around the periphery of the grocery store*: fresh produce, dairy, eggs, and meat. The packaged processed foods are usually in the aisles. So, avoid the aisles unless you need oils, vinegar, nuts and seeds, Dijon mustard, honey, almond or coconut milk, and other single-ingredient products to flavour your dishes.
- *When shopping for produce, use your senses* to decide which fruits and vegetables to buy: gently feel them for freshness and ripeness; smell their fragrance; look at their appearance; taste them, if samples are available. If your senses are excited by what you feel, smell and see, so will your taste buds.
- *Be a "label reader"*: read the ingredient list on packaged food products. Avoid anything containing a long list of weird ingredients that you can't pronounce, or with "lite", "fat-free", "no sugar added" on the label. Most likely, flavouring chemicals have been added to make them more palatable. Instead, choose products that have a short list of ingredients (less than five) that you can recognize as real food.
- *Avoid food products that contain some form of sugar* or sweetener, especially high-fructose corn syrup (HFCS), listed among the top three ingredients.
- *Avoid eating processed foods (food with a list of ingredients)*. I see these foods as *convenience food*. They are not designed to maintain optimal health on a long-term basis. I appreciate their practical usefulness to sustain life in emergency situations when there are limited or no cooking facilities, no refrigeration, and no fresh food available, i.e., a power outage, a storm, a flood, being stranded, etc. As we are experiencing more and more of these emergency situations, it is wise to have available a supply of packaged foods that appeal to you. The rest of the time, we *can* and *should* rely on fresh food from Mother Nature to survive and thrive, just like our ancestors did for millions of years.
- *Spend your grocery money on food that is fresh and live, and has a short expiration da*te.
- If possible, *grow some vegetables* (like tomatoes, lettuce, peppers), and herbs in your backyard or in pots. Enjoy these sun-blessed produce; they can't get fresher than that.

B) Cooking

- To resolve health and weight issues, *cook your own food more often*, making sure that ⅔ of any one meal consist of alkaline foods in the form of a salad, a side dish of raw or cooked vegetables. The other third of the meal is for acidifying foods like meat, fish, and eggs.
- *Food tastes better when it is prepared and presented with loving care*. Whenever you can, put more thought and effort into feeding yourself and your family. There is no activity less selfish and time less wasted than preparing something deliciously nourishing for the people you love. People who cook their own meals with fresh ingredients tend to have a more balanced and healthier nourishment plan because they don't rely on processed food containing excess salt, sugar, fat, and preservatives.

- *If you want to eat, you need to do the two Ps: Plan and Prepare your meals.* Spend a few minutes every day or on a weekly basis to plan what you want to eat, and get the ingredients needed from the grocery store or your freezer. Make the meals big enough so you have enough leftovers for the next day's lunches.
- *To save some time, prepare ahead a few ready-to-go breakfasts and snacks.* For make-ahead ideas, refer to the Breakfast, Snacks and Baking sections of this book and Volume 2.
- *To make meal preparation quicker and easier, you can chop ahead of time the vegetables needed for the next day's recipes,* i.e., salads, soups and stews. Cut the meat, wash the chicken, or shell the shrimp. Refrigerate the prepared ingredients in separate food containers or bags. Putting the meal together will be a breeze.
- *Preparing meals can be a spiritual and mindful activity.* Be patient and present in the moment; do not rush the process. Focus on one task at a time, like chopping onions; then, sweating the onions; allowing the chemical reaction to do its magic. When browning meat, onions or vegetables, take your time to build the flavours created by the caramelizing action as there is a lot of umami (or yummy) flavour in browned food. (After several injuries and mishaps caused by rushing, I learned that being more mindful and slowing down a little makes my cooking experience more enjoyable -- and safer.) Disconnecting for a few minutes or an hour from your work responsibilities, your computer and phone, and reconnecting with your senses, real food, and the people you cook with or for might feel quite therapeutic. You might begin to enjoy cooking.
- *The Chopra Center for Wellbeing says that food is for nourishment.* It recommends using fresh and freshly prepared food whenever possible, as opposed to what is known as *"FLUNC Food"* (Frozen, Leftover, Unnatural, Nuked, Canned). According to Ayurveda (the traditional holistic medical system of India that believes in the importance of the flow of life energy to maintain physical and mental health), food provides more than carbs, proteins, fats, vitamins and trace minerals. It also carries intelligence – life force or *prana* – and the fresher the food, the more life force is available. Frozen or canned foods are not as rich in *prana* as fresh food. However, the Center says that if you can't always find the ideal fresh source, don't worry. How you eat is as important as what you eat. If, while you are preparing and eating your meal, there is joy and love in your heart, the *prana* will be there.
- To make your nourishment plan even more flavourful, *embrace new authentic foods* from ethnic markets, and recipe ideas from cookbooks, magazines, Internet, etc. Spices and fresh herbs add great hypo-caloric flavours to dishes.
- *Choose the best, most flavourful ingredients you can afford.* Great taste and satisfying nourishment don't have to be oxymoronic.
- *Learn new, simple cooking techniques that give great flavour to food* (i.e., poaching, braising). Julia Child said, "You don't have to cook fancy or complicated masterpieces – just good food made from fresh ingredients prepared in a simple way." Let the great flavours of fresh foods satisfy you. Sometimes, only salt and pepper, extra-virgin olive oil and balsamic vinegar are required.
- Using a cooking method of your choice, prepare fresh ingredients to ensure maximum flavour per calorie. *Play with the various tastes: sweet, salty, sour, bitter, spicy-hot, and umami.* The umami taste was first identified by Japanese scientists more than 100 years ago. It often signals edible proteins: all meat, fish, dairy, fruits and vegetables have some protein so they all have some umami. According to Ayurveda, it is beneficial to have all tastes present at every meal. If each taste is blended into a symphony of flavours: 1) the food will be delicious, 2) you will feel satisfied when you have finished eating, and 3) the meal will be nutritionally balanced and complete. I think that when a dish is composed of a well-balanced symphony of flavours, it makes people sing with pleasure!
- *The safest way to cook and heat your food is to use a regular stove or oven.* Numerous studies show that microwaved foods lose 60-90% of their vital energy field. Microwaving alters the food chemistry which can lead to malfunctions in many body systems. It only takes a few more minutes to warm up your leftovers in a regular oven, and cook your meals on the stove. You may notice that the food tastes much better, too. You will be healthier in the long run.
- *Enlist the help of children and other family members in food planning* -- choosing recipes and shopping for the ingredients -- and food preparation to lighten your work. Teaching children how to cook and do chores (like setting the table, cleaning up after dinner, making their lunches for school, putting everything away) is so important for their development as responsible, caring and self-reliant adults. It could be one of the most valuable skills you could teach them. Children who grow up eating flavourful home-cooked meals will more likely help in the kitchen, and cook for themselves; an interest that they will maintain in their adult life, and,

as a result, will keep them in greater health. Also, children who eat home-cooked meals are less likely to be overweight because the portions are smaller than the restaurant's and contain less fat, salt and sugar.

C) Eating

- *If we don't change our habits, the family dinner is about to become a lost ritual.* It should be a time to nourish, converse, laugh and strengthen ties between family members. As frequently as possible, plan, prepare and eat family meals together. Since you spend a significant amount of time and energy cooking, take as much time at the table to enjoy the food, the people and the laughs. Who knows, this supportive family ritual may save your teenager from turning to alcohol, drugs, and dropping out of school.
- *"Dine out" at home*; by creating more healthful and tasty versions of your restaurant favourites at home – whether you are craving Thai, Japanese, French, Greek, or Italian food. You will save money and unnecessary calories. Refer to Part 4 of this book and Part 2 of **Volume 2** for ideas.
- *Sit down at a table to eat* where you feel comfortable, in a relaxing atmosphere, with real plates, glasses and cutlery. If you can't do it every day, create at least one special meal a week i.e., on the weekend when you may have more time. Use real china, music, candles, fresh flowers, and plan an experience that appeals to your senses and nourishes your soul. It lifts the spirits and strengthens family bonds.
- *Before eating, sit down, slow down and take a deep breath.* Remind yourself that it is time to replenish your energies and nourish your body. Bless your food, yourself and your fellow diners before eating. Then, take a moment to place your attention on your food: notice the textures, appreciate the colours, and breathe the aromas reaching your nose. Allow your mouth to salivate in anticipation. It will create a more alkaline environment in your body.
- As much as possible, *take your time to eat*. With your spoon or fork, pick up small amounts of food. Eat slowly by chewing well to liquefy your food with your saliva. As we chew, we generate more saliva which contains enzymes to facilitate the digestion. Enjoy the flavours and the textures in your mouth; it is one of the main reasons why we eat! Between bites, put down your spoon or fork to pause, and allow your stomach to catch up. Then, place your awareness on your stomach to find out if you are full and should stop eating. When you have finished eating, relax and notice how you feel. You should feel relaxed but energized, nourished and satisfied, instead of uncomfortable, stuffed and sleepy.
- *Eat colourful food*, as each colour relates to a gland and a chakra – an energy centre in your body.
- *To control the quality and the amount of salt and sugar, flavour your food yourself.* To season your food, use a pinch of Celtic sea salt, fresh herbs and/or a squirt of citrus juice. Use simple ingredients to craft your own vinaigrettes: oil, vinegar, Dijon mustard, maple syrup or honey. Instead of store-bought sugary dessert, make your own fruit-based treats.
- *It is the first few bites that are the most flavourful and pleasurable.* That is why I like small portions, tapas-style: my satisfaction remains high and my unnecessary calorie intake low.

"He who eats too much knows not how to eat."
-Jean Anthelme Brillat-Savarin,
French jurist and lawyer (1755-1826)

- *Be mindful of your portion sizes.* Use smaller plates, bowls and cups to hold smaller portions of food. And it is quite all right to leave some food on the plate, despite that, while you were growing up, your parents may have told you to eat everything you were served. Ayurveda considers the ideal volume of food to equal about two handfuls as this measure fills most of the stomach, leaving enough space for the food to mix freely with digestive enzymes and *vata* (space and air) energy to push it down through the digestive tract. Wait at least 20 minutes before helping yourself with a second portion.
- In Ayurveda, it is recommended to *follow the meal with digestive enzymes*. In India, as an after-meal ritual, many people munch on a small handful of seeds that assist the digestive process. You can easily create your own blend by mixing in a glass jar equal parts of sesame seeds, fennel seeds and cumin seeds, and keeping it handy in a cool, dry place. To sweeten the breath, mix in a glass jar equal parts of anise seeds, fennel seeds and caraway seeds.
- As much as possible, to improve your digestion, your energy level, and ultimately your health, *be mindful of how you combine your food.* Most protein foods require acid digestive juices produced in the stomach to break

them down, while most carbohydrates require an alkaline fluid produced in the mouth for complete digestion. When the acidic juices mix with the alkaline fluids, they tend to neutralize one another, making the digestion process more difficult and incomplete. How well food is digested also affects the acid/alkaline balance in the body. We all want a more alkaline environment. On a regular basis, enjoy a meal of meat with vegetables, no starchy carbohydrates *or* a meal of vegetables with starchy carbohydrates, no meat. If you want to know more about the rules of proper food combining, there are many books that explain the rules, the principles, the ideal food plan, as well as the good and the not so good food combinations.

- *Before reaching for a snack, ask yourself what you really need at the moment*: is it food, water or fresh air? Often, we mistakenly think we need to eat when in fact we need to hydrate and oxygenate ourselves.
- *When we are bored, we eat mindlessly to entertain ourselves*. Stop eating before you are full so there is enough room in your stomach for the digestion process to take place.
- *Plan your snacks* and take them with you when you leave the house so, when you feel hungry, you are not tempted to eat processed options. Choose natural plant food like nuts and seeds, fruits, raw vegetables, a grain-free muffin (see the **Wholesome and Nourishing Baking** section of this book).
- *There are no bad foods, only bad eating plans lacking nourishment*. Enjoy some of the not so good food as occasional treats. Break the rules once in a while. What matters is what you do *most of the time*. Practice the 85:15 rule -- 85% of the time, cook and eat what your body needs; 15% of the time, enjoy your treats!
- *Cook and eat as though it matters*! Because it does! Your health and your life depend on it.
- *To ensure a restful night of sleep, have a light dinner*. Stop eating at least three hours before bedtime.
- After dinner, instead of watching TV, *go out for a walk with your family*. It helps with the digestion process.

Cooking with the 7 Senses (or my energetic mindset of cooking)

The 5 senses can play an important role in creating a succulent dish that will satisfy your family and guests, and make you burst with pride and joy. Cooking is an organic and experiential activity.

Tasting: You should taste what you are cooking as you proceed down the recipe instructions, if it is appropriate. You don't want to taste raw meat to see how much longer it needs to cook! Tasting the food along the way gives you an idea of what it will be like once the dish is completed. You like it, great! Not quite what you want? You can adjust the seasoning and the flavouring to your personal taste. Make sure you record your modifications in the book.

Seeing: By being visually attentive, you know when an ingredient or a mixture has achieved the desired browning, steaming or whipping for maximum flavour and optimal texture.

Touching: Touching is necessary to gauge the level of ripeness of a fruit or a tomato or an avocado, and the degree of "doneness" of a piece of meat in the pan or on the grill. Don't be afraid to touch your food. That is how you connect with it before it becomes a part of you in your mouth, your stomach, your whole body, your energy. And those of the people you cook for.

Hearing: It tells you when there is a change in chemistry happening in the pot or pan. It often happens when there is a certain amount of moisture involved. Or, for instance, when you roast seeds in a pan and they pop. Paying attention to the "whispering" sounds and the songs the food makes (as my grandmother used to say) while being transformed tells you when you can proceed to the next step.

Smelling: Usually when you start smelling the food being cooked, it means wonderful culinary chemistry is happening. If you are baking something in the oven and you start smelling it, it is almost ready to come out. If you delay too long or ignore the smell, the dish or baked good may be beyond repair. So trust what your nose is sensing way before the smoke detector starts its annoying ear-piercing alarm.

Because the senses, especially smell and sight, can trigger and increase the production of saliva and digestive enzymes, the digestion and assimilation processes begin long before we put any food in our mouth. The so-called "cephalic digestion" (*cephalic* meaning "in the head" in Greek) tells us that the attractive appearance and the pleasing aromas of food promote a more enjoyable eating experience and a better digestion. In other words, *we eat with our eyes and nose first*. I know you would agree that the dining experience is raised to an even higher level when we attractively set the table with good dinnerware, candles, flowers, and relaxing music; and when we share the wonderfully fragrant and appetizing meal with pleasant dining companions.

And finally, two senses that are not often mentioned in cookbooks or in cooking, and, in my opinion, are equally important:

- Your *6th sense* can be of great value and give you your unique "Chef Personality" as you decide intuitively *what* and *how much* to add to your culinary creations, regardless of what the recipe suggests.
- *Cooking from your heart*, whether for your family, your guests or just for yourself, is worth focusing on as it infuses the food you prepare with a distinctive loving quality that can't be measured but can definitely be felt (or tasted) when present, or missed when lacking. The food prepared with love from your heart is more easily absorbed and digested, certainly more enjoyable and memorable. It is filled with greater life force energy; therefore, it is healthier, more nourishing and more life-sustaining than processed, factory-made food, or food prepared in an environment where less than loving feelings were expressed.

So, how do you cook from your heart? By recognizing that the act of cooking, the food, as well as the people you cook for, matter. So much depends on a nourishing, well-balanced, wholesome, satisfying, *and* enjoyable meal. It is often around simple, great-tasting food that the best conversations and exchanges take place, and are remembered.

Since you decided to read this book, I would guess that you are the chosen one whose responsibility is to cook for and feed others. If you can't get yourself to like cooking, you can still infuse the food you prepare with love by using your mind to state a loving intention. As much as you can, put your love and your essence in the food you cook; it is that special one-of-a-kind invisible ingredient that makes your food comforting, nourishing and memorable. The people you feed will keep wanting more of it and be grateful for this expression of love for them.

I look at my role of "the household chef" as an honor, rather than a dreaded chore. Since I am in charge of the cooking and will eat my own creations, I make sure that I cook what I like and infuse my passionate, caring energy into it! You can, too!

Blessings and Thanksgiving

Without being religious, I feel it is a good idea to bless one's meal before eating it to ensure that it is filled with loving energy and intention, and to bless the people who prepared it and those who are about to be nourished with it. Giving thanks before a meal allows us to recognize that many people worked hard to get the food to our table: from the farmers to the grocery store clerks, from the restaurant chef to the friend or relative who transformed the raw food into a delicious dish. Saying grace before a meal reminds us how privileged and fortunate we are to be eating an abundance of fresh, nutritious food on a daily basis.

I have never seen grace being said by people who are rushing around, scarfing down their food, or eating over the sink or in the car; or by people who inhale their meal in five minutes flat. When people say grace at the table (a key piece of furniture *vs.* the couch or the desk or the car seat), they pause … sit still … breathe … create a sacred space for rest and replenishment … and pay attention to what they are about to do: *eat,* instead of just refueling the body. They connect with the food, their bodies and their dining companions, if present. As a result, the main physiological benefit of a pre-meal grace, according to some studies, is mindful and slower eating that improves digestion and assimilation, and gives the body time to register when it is full.

Also, giving thanks before a meal sets the tone at the table as it calms the nerves and tames the spirits. It is pretty hard to argue and fight with our fellow diners after saying grace! Saying grace wherever we are, since it is portable, can elevate a simple meal into an act of re-centering, celebration, and gratitude.

I believe that the nourishment starts in the kitchen, so, I created my own kitchen prayer and posted it on my refrigerator:

Lord, may this kitchen be filled with so much inspired creativity
that preparing the food here is done easily and safely.
May this kitchen be filled with so much peace, joy and love
that everyone who eats the food prepared here feels peaceful, happy and filled with love.
Lord, bless this kitchen and all who cook here.
May who eats the food prepared here receive pleasure, nourishment, and long-lasting wellness.

Intuitive and Enlightened Eating (or my energetic mindset of eating)

Drinking lots of purified water daily is very important for hydration, optimal metabolism and energy. In my opinion, water is the only food that we should ingest every day. All the other foods should be consumed on a rotation basis to avoid the repeated assault of an offensive food on the digestive system, and to prevent developing intolerance, sensitivities and allergies. Also, to maximize our absorption of the necessary vitamins, minerals and antioxidants, it is important to consume a *variety* of water-filled fruits and vegetables, proteins and essential fatty acids, *vs.* the limited favourites.

I have "paleotized" my favourite recipes so they are now gluten-free. And most of them are also dairy- and grain-free. Maximizing the flavours with the freshest ingredients makes me forget about the missing gluten, dairy and grains.

Occasionally, in small amounts, I use some rice, cheese, lentils, and chickpeas in my cooking because I still enjoy these foods, and my body can tolerate them in infrequent small amounts. I gauge my food choices and quantities on the way my body feels. I check in by asking, "What do I feel like eating? What do I need to eat right now?" and wait for an answer. I call that "Intuitive Eating" or "eating with enlightened wisdom". Feeling not too hungry? I don't eat much or delay the meal. Feeling a bit heavy? I drink water, or have a green smoothie or a bowl of clear soup. Feeling tired? I have to admit that this rarely happens now! I drink water, have a green salad; perhaps a few pieces of dried fruit. Sometimes, a walk outside in the sunshine or a power nap is just what I need to perk up.

Speaking of nap, I feel that there is nothing a nap can't fix! When possible, I take a 10- to 20-minute power nap to get an energy boost, some answers about a challenge or clarity when I feel stuck on a project. I wake up feeling energized physically and refreshed mentally with guided inspiration and motivation.

Get in the habit of asking yourself questions. Your Inner-Wise Guide who is directly connected to the Higher Power (or the Divine) knows best and is always on call, waiting to be of service. Don't shush that inner voice: it is who you really are. Trust the answers coming from your Inner-Wise Guide as they are supportive, loving and uplifting. The Ego's answers will not be as supportive; in fact, coming from a lower power, they will be of a rather lower vibration: "Yes, you can have another square of chocolate! Go ahead; you can finish the whole package!" As you get used to eating more real, satisfying, fresh plant-food, your cravings for the not-so-good food will diminish and even disappear, leaving you better able to discern when the Ego's voice is trying to lead you down the wrong path, and when your Inner-Wise Guide is lovingly informing you about more beneficial and nourishing choices.

You have all the answers you need inside of you. All you need to do is ask and wait for them. At first, it can be challenging to notice how these answers are expressed and shared with you as you may not recognize them as the answers you asked for. Your Inner-Wise Guide has its own unique way of communicating with you. Be open and receptive to its communication style.

Why am I mentioning this rather esoteric piece of information in a cookbook?

I strongly believe that, because our levels of energy and health depend mostly on the *quality* and *quantity* of the food, the beverages, and the thoughts we ingest, it is important that we consciously make wise choices. These choices will be reflected in the quality of our lives and, ultimately, in the state of our medical system. Our lives, our performance and our behaviour depend on those choices. And for that, we often need "a second opinion" or a strong recommendation from a reliable source that knows us very well, sometimes better than we know ourselves: our Inner-Wise Guide. I call that "Enlightened Eating". The way I see it, the Inner-Wise Guide is like a combination of a GPS and a compass: it is always ready to steer us in the right direction as we journey on our spiritual path. Connecting with it enables us to tap into our innate intuition and creativity to find answers and solutions to our challenges. If we are open to and aware of the spiritual gifts that we all have, we can even tap into the clairvoyant and clairaudient messages that we receive every day, especially when we ask for assistance and guidance.

Healthy Food and Occasional Treats

In my opinion, what makes a nourishment plan a bad one is when its foundation is not life-sustaining and health-building. The food that we consume each day constitutes our first line of defense against health concerns -- *our immunity*. Good quality food that makes our body vibrant with health and energy is the best medicine, and can assist in the prevention and the healing of health concerns. I think it is important that we have on hand tasty, satisfying and highly nourishing food to minimize cravings and temptations that weaken the body, and to facilitate our efforts to control appetite. It makes more sense to spend the money and the time in prevention now than in treatment and recovery programs later.

The *occasional* treat is quite enjoyable and doesn't threaten the whole body's wellness. I believe that by indulging in the occasional treats in moderation is so much healthier (and more fun) than coming from a mindset of denial, deprivation and restriction. There is no need to feel guilty about occasional indulgences; the key words must be *occasional* and *planned*. In fact, it is a good idea to include *some* (not all of them) of your favourite treats in your nourishment plan and decide when and how much you are *planning* on eating. When you have a treat, slow down! Take your time to savour it, using all your senses: notice its appearance, smell its fragrance, touch its texture and temperature, place a small amount on your tongue and let it linger there... then ... when you are ready to eat it, notice the texture under your teeth and feel your taste buds explode with enjoyment! Listen to the sound that the food makes in your mouth as you slowly eat it. Take a moment to notice how your whole being feels from enjoying the treat. Savoring a small piece of chocolate this way – if chocolate is your weakness that gives you unspeakable bliss -- could take 10 minutes or more! The benefit: you are totally aware, mindful, satisfied -- and pleased that you are not overdoing it!

> *"Most people would like to be delivered from temptation but would like to keep in touch."*
> -Robert Orben, U.S. humorist

When you have planned a treat in your meal plan, your body and your spirit will feel satisfied instead of deprived and punished; and there will be no need to sneak in any unhealthy food to satisfy a craving, and as a result, feel guilty. The same goes for any leisure activity or anything you see as "treats": include them in your day or week, take your time to enjoy them and notice how you feel. I think that the occasional treats should be seen as "fun entertainment food" in a *"fun-*damentally" supportive nourishment plan. They are part of a well-balanced life. You decide on the frequency and the quantity.

However, if there are 'treat' foods that you really don't want to eat, or shouldn't eat because they make you ill, you know that succumbing to the temptation is not worth it: you experience a setback. It is wise to avoid bringing these foods in the house or your environment. If someone brings them in your environment, especially in your home, request that the "offensive" food be hidden from you so you can more easily avoid temptation and the sabotaging of your best efforts.

When we pay attention to the guidance that we receive after asking for it and we take appropriate actions, our cooking and eating become enlightened and healthier. No need to count calories. It becomes easier to enjoy food as it is meant to be enjoyed, savoured and appreciated. Eating real food is a pleasure that should be fully enjoyed as it nourishes not only the body but the mind-brain and the soul, too. After eating, we should be feeling good and happy as opposed to ill, bloated and guilty.

Why We Should Spend More Time in the Kitchen

As I mentioned before, in order to be healthier as individuals and as a nation, we need to spend more time in the kitchen cooking the food we need to eat.

As the home chef, with my care, my creative passion and my vibration, I can magically transform simple ingredients into synergistic life-sustaining and health-building delights. (It is not a special gift; just a passionate motivation.) I am aware of the relationships I have with the plants and the meat that I cook, the earth, the farmers and their values, my heritage, my culture, Philip's culture and others because I like to cook international cuisines, my values, my food memories, and the people my cooking nourishes, pleases and inspires.

When you walk in a home, there is nothing more welcoming than a wonderful food aroma greeting you from the kitchen. Cooking connects us and brings us together. Appetizing food aromas lift our spirit, put a smile on our face and make our mouth salivate. We suddenly become happy, anticipating what will be served. Cooking and sharing meals at the table together are the most important activities that we can do as families to improve our health and our home life. It's a concrete, hands-on activity that requires creative imagination and co-operation. It makes us happy. I know my heart is bursting with joy and excitement when I prepare a new dish and I can't wait for Philip to taste it. Then, I can't wait for him to tell me what he thinks. Sometimes, I have to encourage him to like it! But that doesn't stop me from creating new recipes because nothing pleases me more than someone – especially Philip or a child – *ooohing* and *aaahing* with delight. I feel honor and joy when they request that I make it again and again.

Cooking is a great way to connect with children and especially teenagers, to remind them again of social skills they may have forgotten -- such as table manners, listening, taking turns, engaging in conversations without being unpleasant, making eye contact and refraining from texting. Cooking our own meals is important to help improve our eating habits and lifestyle, to make them healthier and more life-sustaining for generations to come. Our current and future health, as well as the sustainability of our medical system, depends on it.

Being able to cook is one of the basic survival skills to have. I feel sorry for many adults, young and not so young, who don't know how to put a meal together without a microwave oven, packaged food or restaurant take-out. I know that spending more time cooking in the *gathering room* of the house -- the kitchen -- will reduce our time spent in the emergency *waiting room* of the hospital. It's time to regain control of our cooking and see it as a "cool" and fun activity that brings enjoyment, encourages sharing and develops self-sufficiency. Otherwise, I fear that, in a few years, cooking a meal with real ingredients will be seen as exotic and a lost art, even though we seem fascinated by the cooking shows on television. Home-cooked food matters. It is filled with life force and love. It should be part of a happy and vibrant life. By allowing ourselves to make wiser choices regarding what we nourish our bodies with, we begin to reclaim our health and our power.

Celebrating Our Cultural Diversity

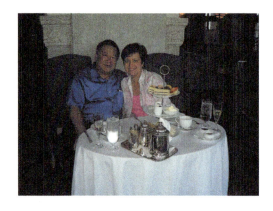

This cultural diversity is present in my household: Philip is Canadian-born Chinese, and I am Canadian-born French. Our Franco-Chinese Fusion has been feeding my interest in Mediter-asian cuisine ever since we started sharing our lives together. *(Photo of Philip and I enjoying an afternoon tea experience in Banff, Alberta. Gluten-free options are available almost everywhere now.)*

I love traveling. Without leaving my kitchen, I can transport myself to other countries by combining ingredients that release exotic aromas and flavours. The collection of gluten-free, Paleo spa recipes in this book and in **Volume 2** is an invitation for you to explore the diverse cuisines by joining me on a journey through the Mediterranean and the Asian regions, without jetlag.

Using this book, you, the home cook, can find something to ignite your creative imagination with:

- your current kitchen equipment,
- your food memories from your cultural background,
- the fresh produce available in your area.

The following recipes are only suggestions. Feel free to modify the ingredient list and the techniques to suit your palate, equipment and creativity. I hope you will find these recipes appetizing, approachable and, most importantly, nourishing. I also hope you will enjoy this book as much as I have enjoyed creating it with you in mind. It came to form from:

- my love of great food from Mother Nature,
- the desire to cook more creatively and intuitively with a light touch rather than with fuss and exact measuring,
- the concern I have for the numerous individuals who are, unfortunately, experiencing health and weight issues caused by a lack of proper nourishment and guidance, and
- the love of the people I cook for.

Remember ...

Allow Mother Nature to inspire your dinner and nourish YOU! Decide to enjoy and appreciate the abundance of fresh produce, quality meats, oils, nuts, seeds, and the wonderful flavours of the world, rather than focus on the foods that you can't (or shouldn't) eat. Go to your kitchen, put on your apron, and pull out your chef's knife and cutting board. Follow the recipes in this book and create simple but scrumptious spa meals that will easily transform your health – and your life -- for the better. You and your family will feel nourished, satisfied and healthier.

Part 4- Creating Your Own "EMaSC"--
Your Everyday Mediter-asian Spa Cuisine to Nourish Mind, Body and Spirit During Your Spa Care Ritual and Every Day After

Please note that none of the recipes in this book contain: wheat, yeast, gluten, peanut, grain, corn, GMO soy, refined sugar.

To replace the soy sauce in Asian dishes, I recommend using very small amounts of organic wheat-free Tamari sauce made with organic non-GMO soy beans. Some recipes call for full fat, organic dairy in the form of butter, cheese, cream or plain yogurt. For many of these recipes, the dairy is optional.

The preparation and cooking times are approximate depending on your cooking skills, kitchen equipment and environment. You may need to add 5-10 minutes, or more, to the suggested times, especially the first time you experiment with a recipe. To avoid rushing, getting frustrated and injuring yourself, allow yourself extra time to cook.

To ensure successful cooking sessions with minimal to no aggravation at all, here is what I strongly suggest,

1. *Look at cooking as a fun craft project* that will give you an edible and tasty art piece at the end.
2. As you would for any recipe in other cookbooks, *read the whole recipe* you are interested in *before starting to cook.*
3. *Assemble all the required ingredients, supplies, and kitchen equipment.* If you are missing 1 or 2 ingredients and can do without or can replace them with different ones, great! You can proceed with the *mise en place* (cutting and measuring all ingredients and keeping them in prep bowls or plates, ready for a smooth cooking and assembling process. This important step in food preparation can be done several hours ahead; cover and refrigerate the prep bowls.) If you can't modify the recipe, choose another one that lists the ingredients you currently have on hand. Remember, the recipes are only guidelines. Feel free to write on sticky notes or directly in the book your own modifications for the recipes that you experiment with. The dishes you prepare will be amazing and truly nourishing when you infuse them with your creative passion, your intuition, and your personal loving touch.
4. *Wear an apron to protect your clothes.* I have ruined enough tops to know that I need one, not because I am a messy cook, but because unexpected splashes and stains can ruin a top I like. I see my apron as the kitchen uniform that I put on before I pull out my knives, cutting board and prep bowls. My whole being, at a cellular level, knows that I am about to do some serious playing with food! It feels like something is missing when I start preparing food without wearing it, just like sitting in the car or an airplane seat and not buckling up. Also, to be able to stand comfortably for long periods of time, when I am cooking up a storm, I always wear a pair of indoor shoes; otherwise I tend to get sore feet and legs.
5. *Being comfortable* in what we do and finding enjoyment in it is important as that energy of comfort and enjoyment is transferred to our work and, by extension, to the food we cook. Otherwise, no comfort or enjoyment: why bother? So, relax, be mindful of each slice of knife, of each swirl of spoon, of each sample tasting. Enjoy the process of cooking and the magic that will manifest from your loving efforts.

Most of the spa recipes that follow can be prepared in less than 30-45 minutes. Some recipes like the classic *Osso buco,* and the *coq au vin* require more preparation and cooking time to develop maximum flavours and become delicious, comforting soul food. They are great weekend projects or when you have a few free hours. You know that, once the dish is performing its magic in the pot, you are free to do other things. Just check on it once in a while and follow your nose.

I look forward to joining you in your kitchen, through this nourishment-for-wellness book open on your counter, guiding you through the tasty nourishing meal ideas that follow. I know you will be pleased with your spa dishes, and so will the people you cook for. Are you ready to put on your apron and pull out your cutting board and knife? Let's get cooking!

Here is my **Nourishment-for-wellness Formula** for a healthy and happy life:

Honest Decluttering
+ Wise Shopping
+ Intuitive Cooking
+ Mindful Eating
+ Regular Home Spa Rejuvenating
___

Vibrant Living!

"Vibrant health, happiness and longevity come to those
who enjoy cooking and sharing real food with family and friends."
- Marie-Claire Bourgeois, Mediter-asian nourishment foodie

Starting the Day

Breakfast

The most important meal of the day as it "breaks the fast".
It can be nutritious, quick and easy to prepare; or a more elaborate, sit-down, no-hurry meal to splurge with the family on the weekend. One thing is for sure, we should start the day with *real food*, not refined or processed.
Something delicious and nourishing that will fuel us mentally and physically to face the day ahead.
As a child, I didn't like food, and breakfast was the meal I dreaded the most to eat: I was *never* hungry.
I could not bring myself to eat anything.
I often went to school still fasting, despite my mother's effort to make me eat what she had prepared for me. When I moved out on my own, I started bringing breakfast (sometimes more than one) with me
so I could eat it when I was hungry in class or at work.
What still works today is starting slowly, shortly after I get up, with "Breakfast Part 1"
consisting of a bowl of fresh fruits with nuts and spices;
then, ½ hour to 1½ hours later, moving to a more substantial and sustaining "Part 2".
I know that when I eat breakfast, I am not too famished by lunch time,
and I don't crave stuff I am not supposed to eat throughout the day.
Also, my metabolism remains steady, my performance near optimal,
and my disposition, well, I must admit, more agreeable!
I tend to get cranky and impatient when I don't eat enough.
So much depends on eating good food in the right amount, and, for me, at the right time,
so I can remain adorable.
I hope that the following recipes will inspire you to make breakfast and take the time to enjoy it,
preferably sitting down, wherever you take it.

Quick and Portable Breakfast Ideas

- Hard-boiled eggs
- Homemade hot vegetable soup
- Steamed vegetables (perhaps leftover from the supper before)
- Any suggestion from the **Snacks and Beverages** section that appeals to you.
- An open-face sandwich made with any bread recipes from the **Wholesome and Nourishing Baking** section, covered with an avocado spread or a tapenade or a topping of roasted tomatoes, arugula and Parmesan.

Exotic Fruit Salad

Serves 4
Prep Time: 10 min.

This pretty salad allows you to be as creative as you want with the fruit you have on hand.
It makes a wonderful "breakfast appetizer" or a healthy no-baking-required dessert.
It can be packed to go.

Zest and juice of 1 lime
Seeds of ½ pomegranate☺
1 mango, peeled, pitted and chopped
½ pineapple, chopped
3 kiwis, peeled and sliced
12 lychees, canned or fresh and peeled
1 cup of grapes, red, green or blue, seeded
Fresh mint sprig, chopped

1. Add lime zest and juice to a large mixing bowl. Stir to blend.
2. Add the fruit pieces. Stir gently to coat. Sprinkle with chopped mint.
3. Divide in serving bowls and serve. If it is for dessert, serve it in pretty glassware, topped with black sesame seeds.

Variations:

- Add ¼ cup of toasted nuts such as almonds, pine nuts.
- Add 1-2 tbsp of ground flaxseeds and 1 tbsp of flaxseed oil.
- For garnish, add 1-2 tbsp toasted sesame seeds or black sesame seeds or a combination.
- Add 1 tsp finely grated ginger, or candied ginger.
- Instead of mint, thinly sliced basil and coriander leaves give this salad a Thai essence.

☺For a demonstration on how to extract the "juicy rubies" out of a pomegranate, visit my website www.olivestolychees.com

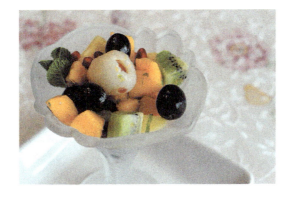

French-style Scrambled Eggs

Serves 4
Prep Time: 5 min.
Cooking Time: 5-8 min.

I was inspired by Laura Calder,
a Canadian cookbook author and host of Food Network Canada's series *French Food at Home*,
to create my version of these delicious easy-to-prepare eggs.
You will like this simple dish for breakfast, lunch or even as a light dinner.
You can omit the cheese if you prefer a dairy-free version.

4 eggs
1 tbsp butter or ghee or coconut oil
Black pepper
Optional: 2-3 tbsp Boursin☺ or grated parmesan
A choice of fresh chopped herbs: chives, parsley, basil, chervil, dill or thyme

1. Separate the eggs in 2 bowls. In the 1st bowl, with a fork, beat the whites a little bit.
2. In the 2nd bowl, beat the yolks with the pepper, cheese (if using) and herbs.
3. Melt the butter or oil in a small pan over medium-low heat. Swirl the melting butter all over the bottom and the sides of the pan. Pour in the whites, and cook over low heat, stirring constantly with a wooden spoon, scraping the sides and bottom of the pan until the egg whites start to turn white and cloudy.
4. Add the yolk mixture; keep cooking and stirring until they combine, but the mixture remains a moist mass.
5. Remove from heat. Serve with some steamed vegetables or a green salad. You can also serve it with gluten-free toasts rubbed with a clove of garlic.

☺*Boursin* is a fresh soft cheese found at the supermarket. It comes in a variety of flavours. I like it because it is very versatile, it has a creamy texture that can easily be blended in a mixture, and it is made with real ingredients such as milk and cream, bacterial cultures, garlic, salt and pepper, herbs. It can be spread over crackers or cucumber rounds. A small amount goes a long way.

*Did you know that, for maximum freshness,
eggs should be stored with the pointed end down?*

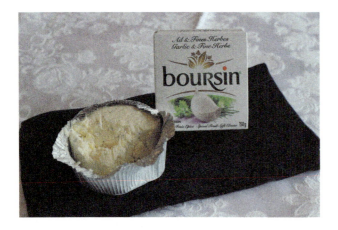
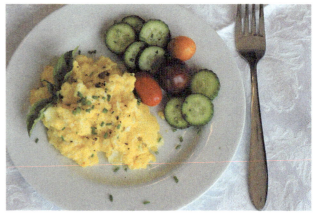

Spanish Tortilla

Serves 4
Prep Time: 20 min.
Cooking Time: 20-25 min.

1-1½ lb potatoes, peeled and thinly sliced
3-4 tbsp olive or coconut oil
1 large onion, thinly sliced
1 garlic clove, minced
6-8 large eggs, lightly whisked

½ tsp each of Celtic salt, black pepper and red pepper flakes
Chopped parsley for garnish
Optional: ½-inch cubes or thin strips of ham, and chopped roasted red pepper for a little sweetness

1. Preheat oven to 400°F. Place potato slices in a large saucepan and cover with cold water. Bring to a boil and cook until tender, about 2-3 minutes. Drain; let cool.
2. Pour the oil in a large non-stick, ovenproof pan over medium-high heat. Add the onion and cook until translucent. Add garlic and potato slices. Add the ham and the red peppers, if using. Cook until golden brown for 4-5 minutes, stirring occasionally. Season with salt, pepper and pepper flakes.
3. Lower the heat and pour in the whisked eggs. Cook without stirring for 4-6 minutes or until the edges are firm. Carefully transfer pan to oven, and bake for 4-6 minutes, or until the eggs are set and slightly golden.
4. Cut into wedges and garnish with parsley. Serve with a green salad or steamed vegetables.

Egg Crêpes

Makes approx. 12 crêpes, depending on your pan size
Prep Time: 5 min.
Cooking Time: 10-15 min.

Inspired by a Chinese cooking show I once saw on television, I make these easy and versatile wheat-free crêpes often. These crêpes can be savory or sweetened for dessert. Also, when cut in thin strips, they can replace egg noodles in a soup or chicken broth. Just roll each crêpe and slice into thin fettuccine of about ½ inch wide. Add to the hot broth with chopped parsley just before serving.

2-3 tbsp butter or coconut oil
6-7 eggs, lightly beaten with some Celtic salt and pepper

1. On medium heat, warm up a non-stick frying pan or a crêpe pan if you have one.
2. Place approximately ½ tbsp or less of butter and warm it up. Rotate the pan to evenly coat the bottom with the melted butter. Ladle a thin layer of crêpe batter in the pan, rotating the pan to coat the bottom and sides evenly.
3. When the batter bubbles in the middle, with a spatula, gently lift the crêpe and turn it over. Cook for a few seconds on the other side.
4. When cooked, slide the crêpe out of the pan onto a large plate. Cover each crêpe with a paper towel so the next crêpe you make doesn't stick to the previous one. Repeat the process with the rest of the batter.
5. **Filling:** Place a crêpe on a cutting board. Lay the filling off centre of the crêpe. Roll the crêpe from one end to the other. You can cut it in thirds or leave it whole.

Suggestions for filling:

- **Savory filling:** To add extra flavour you can include some of the following ingredients. <u>Vegetables</u>: stir-fried mushrooms and onion slices, steamed asparagus. <u>Meat</u>: cooked chicken pieces or ham, grilled shrimp or beef. <u>Herbs</u>: parsley, coriander, chives. <u>Spices</u>: curry powder, ground coriander and ginger.
- **Sweet filling:** Strawberries, bananas, slices of peaches or nectarines, pineapple pieces, topped with whipped cream or drizzled with a chocolate sauce. **Note**: if you want *a dessert crêpe*, you may want to sweeten the batter with 1-2 tsp of cane sugar, maple syrup or sucanat. You can even flavour it with some cocoa powder, cinnamon or vanilla.

Create-Your-Own Breakfast Cereal

Serves 2
Prep Time: 15 min.

For many people, breakfast cereal consisting of flakes tossed unceremoniously in a bowl and covered with several glugs of milk is a regular morning staple. It is often a meal that is mindlessly scarfed down while performing other tasks while getting ready to leave the house. With a little creativity, we can handcraft our own healthy grain-free mix and elevate this meal to something that has great eye and taste buds appeal, is nourishing, and that we look forward to. Mix it all up and see which blend will become your favourite. After all, we eat with our eyes first, and breakfast is – supposedly – the most important meal of the day. (I say all meals are important; otherwise, it is not fair to lunch and dinner!)

The Secret? There is no recipe! Out of the following elements, choose what you like to build your own handcrafted powerful, high-fiber blend with various colours and textures, keeping in mind that single, unprocessed ingredients are the best.

The Base -- Nuts and Seeds: They add protein and provide a good dose of heart-healthy mono-unsaturated fat to help boost the HDL (or good) cholesterol while lowering the LDL (bad) cholesterol. Create your own combination with the following: almonds, walnuts, pine nuts, Brazilian nuts, macadamia, cashews, flaxseeds, pumpkin seeds, sunflower seeds, sesame seeds (light and dark), hemp seeds, chia seeds (white and dark), etc.

Fruits: Scatter a few pieces of fresh and/or dried fruits of your choice: banana, apple or pear chunks, berries, mango, kiwi, goji berries, mulberries, golden berries (or ground cherries), figs, cherries, coconut flakes, etc.

Superfoods: They contain high levels of antioxidants, vitamins and minerals. I like the superfoods from *Organic Traditions*. Use about a teaspoon or so of what you can find and afford: chlorella powder, lucuma powder, spirulina powder, maca powder, camu camu powder, etc. These products can be found in most natural health stores.

Flavouring: Ground spices like cinnamon, cloves, cardamom; vanilla extract; cacao nibs (for a mild natural chocolate flavour; doesn't that make breakfast more interesting?); candied ginger; bee pollen; fresh mint leaves.

The Milk: Coconut or almond, or other nut milk.

To save some time, you can store portions of your dry crafted blend in glass jars, and when ready for breakfast, transfer to a bowl, add fresh fruits and milk.

For a portable breakfast, pack the cereal in a container and the milk in a thermos. You are ready for a great day!

"Love lights more fires than hate extinguishes."
-Ella Wheeler Wilcox

Spiced Applesauce

Makes 1 quart
Prep Time: 10-15 min.
Cooking Time: 20-25 min.

Delicious warm or at room temperature, you and the kids in your life will like this cooked applesauce. If you choose to purée it, the consistency and flavour are quite similar to the store-bought version. Very versatile, this sauce can be part of breakfast with the grain-free granola, a snack with some chopped nuts, or even a dessert with a spoonful of yogurt. You can also use it as a filling for egg crêpes, and a topping for a pork dish. The **Egg Crêpes** recipe is in this section.

Feel free to modify the amount of spices. Personally, I like the applesauce to have noticeable spicy flavour, chai-like. (Chai is a fragrant and delicious Indian tea made with warm spices.) Just remember how much of each whole spice you add to the pot so it is easy to remove all of them once the apples are cooked.

8 apples, peeled, cored and cut into chunks. (Any apple type or combination of apples will work well. Use what you have in the refrigerator.) For a slight pink tint, I add a few of the bright red peels to the saucepan.
2 tbsp butter or ghee
3 tbsp water
½ vanilla bean, split lengthwise, or 1 tsp vanilla extract

1 cinnamon stick
2 star anise
10 whole cloves
1 small piece of fresh gingerroot
10 cardamom pods
A strip of orange rind, as long as you like
2-3 tbsp cane sugar or sucanat or coconut sugar

1. Put the apple chunks, the butter and the water in a heavy saucepan. Add the vanilla bean, the spices and the orange rind, and the sugar. Simmer over medium-low heat until the apples are completely tender and have cooked to a rough purée, stirring them gently from time to time, about 20-25 minutes.
2. Taste the sauce for sweetness, add more sugar if you find it too tart.
3. Remove from heat and set aside to cool. Discard the vanilla bean, the spices and the orange rind before serving. I like to purée the sauce with a hand-held blender for a creamy, smooth consistency.
4. Refrigerate the unused portion. It can keep for about 1 week.

Did you know that cinnamon comes from the inner bark of a tropical Ceylon evergreen tree?

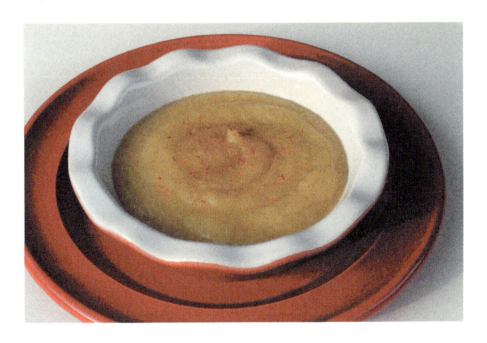

While Waiting for the Next Meal

Snacks and Beverages

Since I have embarked on this gluten-free lifestyle, I have noticed that I no longer need an afternoon snack to tie me over to dinner. That means I need less calories and my body is working more efficiently on the nourishment it receives. It frees me to concentrate on more important things, other than debate how I could satisfy nagging hunger pangs or a relentless craving. If you are now living without gluten yourself, perhaps you have made the same pleasant observation.

Should you need, on occasion, a little extra energy to carry on, following are a few suggestions for healthy snacks and beverages that are plant-food based. If you need to have a snack, or something to substantiate your breakfast, here are some options that are quick, nutritious and filling:

- a cup of apple sauce with ½ tsp cinnamon, 1 tsp ground flaxseeds and some almonds (ground or whole)
- apple wedges topped with almond butter, cinnamon, orange zest and a sprinkle of ground flaxseeds
- a cup of green tea (for some reason, I find a cup of hot liquid quite filling)
- a handful of olives, cherry tomatoes and walnuts or almonds
- a cup of hot homemade broth (vegetable, or chicken and vegetables)
- celery and carrot sticks with tapenade or avocado spread
- a small smoothie with berries and greens
- a handful of nuts and dried fruit
- banana pieces dipped in seeds.

And sometimes, I treat myself to a piece of dark chocolate that I let melt and linger in my mouth!
A piece of heaven!

*"The secret of health for both mind and body is not to mourn for the past,
not to worry about the future, or not to anticipate troubles,
but to live the present moment wisely and earnestly."*
--Buddha

Satisfying Trail Mix

Makes 3¼ cups
Prep Time: 15 min.
Cooking Time: 30-40 min.

Here is a delicious option for a healthy afternoon snack. You can use whatever nut and dried fruit you like and have on hands. Be creative with the combination and quantity of nuts and dried fruit, as well as the spices. You can craft a different batch each time. With some coconut or almond milk, this can make a nice and sustaining Paleo cereal option.

½ cup raw pecans
½ cup raw cashews
½ cup raw almonds
¼ cup sunflower seeds
¼ cup pumpkin seeds
¼ cup maple syrup
1 tsp vanilla extract
¼ tsp ground cinnamon
¼ tsp ground nutmeg

¼ tsp ground ginger
⅛ tsp ground cloves
Pinch of Celtic salt
¼ dried cranberries
¼ cup candied ginger, finely chopped
¼ cup dried goji berries
¼ cup dried cherries
¼ cup dried mango, chopped

1. Preheat the oven to 350°F. Line a baking sheet with a piece of parchment paper.
2. Place nuts on the paper in a single layer. Roast 10-12 minutes, turning once until the nuts are fragrant. Keep an eye on them to prevent burning! Remove from the oven and set aside in a mixing bowl.
3. Reduce the oven to 300°F. Combine the syrup, vanilla, spices and salt in a saucepan. Heat over medium-high until boiling point. Remove the saucepan from the heat and drizzle the syrup over the mixed nuts. Stir well to coat.
4. Spread the nuts back onto the lined baking sheet in a single layer. Bake for 20-25 minutes. Remove the mixture from the oven and let cool completely.
5. Once cool, add the dried fruit; toss to combine. Store in an airtight container for up to 2 weeks.

Did you know that ginger was the first Indian spice known in Europe?

Nutritious Beverages

A-Water

Good quality water should be the main daily beverage for proper hydration of the whole body and brain; improved metabolism; increased energy level; smooth and more fluid joints; improved quality of sleep, and optimal overall wellness.

To make plain water more interesting to drink or when you want to infuse a natural flavour, without any calories, you can add any of the following in a clear glass pitcher, fill with fresh water and allow the flavours to infuse in the refrigerator:

- a few freshly cut and squeezed lemon, orange or lime wedges, with a small sprig of rosemary or lemon verbena;
- orange slices with peeled ginger slices;
- fresh mint sprigs, lemon slices and peeled ginger slices;
- fresh coriander sprigs with lime slices;
- a few cucumber slices with fresh mint leaves;
- a few pieces of berries;
- slices of other fruits like strawberries, peaches or melon;
- sprigs of fresh mint and lemon verbena or lemon balm.

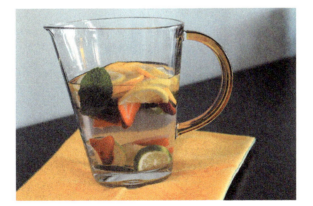

B-Green Tea and Tisanes

Green tea is also a great beverage choice, low in caffeine, high in antioxidants. Studies have shown that *matcha*, a very fine powder made from the youngest top leaves of the tea plant, is the healthiest beverage on the planet because the entire tea leaf is consumed. Because it contains Nature's highest source of L-theanine (an amino acid that provides balanced sustained energy and increases alpha production in the brain) and catechins, it provides the consumer with approximately 10 times more of the health-promoting nutrient of steeped green tea. With an ORAC (*Oxygen Radical Absorbance Capacity: a measurement of the antioxidant capacities of different foods*) of 4,000 per teaspoon serving (or 3 g), matcha provides the highest level of protective antioxidant, making it the greatest of the superfoods. You can add a small amount (½ - 1 tsp) to a smoothie.

A bowl or cup of matcha

In a matcha bowl or mug, blend ½ tsp of matcha and a small amount of hot water. With a spoon or a traditional bamboo, whisk to make a smooth paste. Add more water to fill the bowl or cup. You can also add ½ tsp of honey, if you like. To avoid scorching the precious green matcha powder, the ideal water temperature is between 65-85°C/160-185°F. To achieve the ideal temperature range, boil some water and let it stand for 6-8 minutes. For a demonstration on how to prepare a delicious bowl of matcha, visit my website at www.olivestolychees.com.

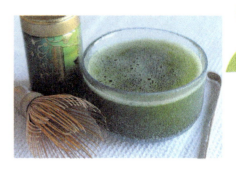

Moroccan Mint Tea

Mint tea, the national sweet drink and the essence of Moroccan hospitality, is offered throughout the day in people's homes, in cafés and restaurants, and at the end of a meal. Prepared by brewing Chinese gunpowder (or loose green tea leaves), with a generous handful of fragrant mint sprigs and large amounts of sugar, it is then poured from a height to aerate the tea into decorated glasses. It is served to quench the thirst even on a hot day and to aid digestion after a meal.

1-1½ tbsp Chinese gunpowder or green tea leaves
A large handful of fresh mint sprigs
4-5 tsp of coconut sugar or the sweetener of your choice

Pour some boiling water into the teapot to warm it, swirling the water around. Pour it out. Put tea, mint and sugar in the pot. Pour boiling water over the contents. Stir the tea until the mint starts floating to the surface and the sugar has dissolved. Allow about 5 minutes to infuse.

Arrange 4 to 6 tea glasses close to one another. Hold the teapot just above the first glass. As you pour, raise the teapot higher to create a little froth on the surface. Continue with the other glasses. Enjoy the tea on its own or with some desserts.

*"Women are like tea bags;
we don't know our true strength until we are in hot water."*
-Eleanor Roosevelt

Lover's Tea Blend

I love this sensual tea made with fragrant herbs and spices. I use the herbs from my garden. The ingredients can be found at the grocery store and at a farmers' market. Use what you have and it will taste great.

2 whole cloves
2 star anise
2-3 cardamom pods
½ cup lemon verbena or lemon
balm leaves (dried or fresh)

¼ cup lavender
¼ cup dried rose petals (I find them in packages in the tea aisle of Asian grocery stores.)
2 tbsp mint leaves

Use a spice grinder or a mortar and pestle to crush the spices to a coarse powder. Transfer to a mixing bowl. Add the rest of the ingredients and mix well. Keep in a covered container in a dark and cool place.

To make tea for 2: Bring 3 cups of water to a boil. Warm up a teapot with some of the hot water by swirling the water around inside. Discard the water. Place 1 tbsp of Lover's Tea Blend in the teapot and cover with boiled water. Steep for a few minutes and serve immediately. Serve with some fresh strawberries.

Lemon Mint Ginger Tisane

I like this drink when I want something comforting with a digestive boost.

4 cups of boiling water
3 slices of lemon, with some grated zest
1 slice (or to taste) of ginger, peeled and grated
1 sprig of fresh mint
1 tsp honey, optional

In a teapot, mix the ingredients together, squishing the lemon slices and bruising the mint leaves. Steep for a few minutes and discard the mint leaves.

I-have-a-cold-and-I-don't-feel-too-well Comfort Tea

This old-fashioned concoction, full of medicinal properties, is pleasant to the palate, the stomach and the whole being. Its pungent and spicy flavours have been a favored treatment for centuries. The ginger has warming properties and the ability to calm an upset stomach, while the lemon's fragrance lifts the spirit.

4 cup hot water
5-6 star anise
A handful of fresh or dried mint or spearmint
1 tsp whole cloves
1-2 tsp lemon and orange zest or a large strip cut from the peel without the white pith
1 slice of ginger, peeled (it can also be grated)
5-6 cardamom pods
1 tsp honey (optional)

Bring the water to a boil. Place the ingredients in a teapot large enough to hold the 4 cups of water. Pour the hot water over the herbs and spices. Allow to steep for 5 minutes. Pour yourself a mugful, relax, breathe deeply, and enjoy. Do something fun or do nothing. You probably got sick because you are doing too much! So, have a hot bath and go to bed. I mean it! Refer to **Volume 2** for suggestions on the **Art of Feeling Well**.

Alkaline Morning Tonic

This tonic, from Nonpareil, a spa facility near Toronto, is taken on an empty stomach. It is a delicious drink that helps alkalize the body, stimulate the bowels, and boost the circulatory system. Mix the following ingredients together in a cup.

1 cup of hot water
Juice of 1 lemon
1 tbsp maple syrup
1 tbsp apple cider vinegar, organic and unpasteurized
1 pinch or more of cayenne pepper

According to the spa facility, the apple cider vinegar helps to cleanse the body of toxic wastes while improving digestion and strengthening the heart. It is recommended for arthritic conditions because the uric acid crystals tend to collect in the bursa (small serous sac between a tendon and a bone) and joints of the body resulting in bursitis and arthritis. To flush the uric acid crystals, it is recommended to take 1-2 tsp of apple cider vinegar with 1-2 tsp raw honey in a glass of distilled water, 3 times a day. It helps make the joints more elastic and flexible.

C- Smoothies and Blended Beverages

The following beverages are easy and very quick to make. They are surprisingly filling, thanks in part to the fibrous pulp. They are portable in a thermos or a bottle designed for cold drinks. I use a blender like NutriBullet® (a high-powered blender from the maker of The Magic Bullet). A regular blender works well, too. To fit your blender, feel free to reduce some of the ingredient amounts. Taste and adjust the flavours to your liking. Most of these recipes make 1 large serving or 2 small ones, if you *have* to share.

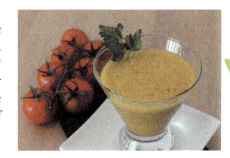

Note: To activate the digestive enzymes in the saliva of your mouth, before swallowing, swirl and "chew" several times each mouthful of juice or smoothie. When chewing, the food becomes coated with enzymes in the saliva that help break it down, speed up the digestion process, and allow greater absorption of nutrients. Take your time and savour the flavours.

A Liquid Soup for Lunch

In a blender, combine until smooth:

- 3 medium tomatoes, cut into chunks
- 1 cup carrot juice (preferably organic)
- ½ cup water
- 1 tbsp balsamic vinegar
- 1 tbsp extra-virgin olive oil
- 2 tsp organic tamari
- 1 small garlic clove
- A pinch of cayenne pepper
- A few strands of fresh chives
- Fresh leaves of basil, coriander and parsley.
- Save a few for garnishing, if desired.

Variation: For a creamy version, you can add half an avocado. You can also add half a cucumber or a few leaves of spinach or kale for extra green power.

Pep-To-Cu

In a blender, combine until smooth:

½ red **Pep**per, seeded and cut in pieces, 2 large **To**matoes, cored and cut in pieces, ½ English **Cu**cumber, peeled and cut in pieces, 1 small **garlic clove**, chopped, 1 tsp **lemon juice**, a few leaves of **fresh spinach, parsley, coriander, mint and basil.**

Make-Me-Feel-Better Drink

In a blender, combine until smooth and then strain:

1 cup of **orange juice**, 1 small piece of **cucumber**, peeled (about 2 inches), 1 cup of **tomato juice** or vegetable juice like V8, **fresh chives, parsley, basil**

Serve immediately.

Green Power Drink

In a blender, combine until smooth:

1 Granny Smith **apple**, cored, quartered, 1 tbsp **lemon juice** or 2 tbsp **orange juice**, a 4-inch piece of English **cucumber**, ½ cup each of **kale and spinach**, chopped, 1 cup **romaine lettuce**, chopped, a handful of **parsley leaves**, a thin slice of **fresh ginger**, ½ tsp **chlorella or spirulina**, water as needed.

Detox Blend

In a blender, combine until smooth:

1 **beet**, peeled and cut in small pieces, 1 **celery stalk**, cut in pieces, 1 **apple**, cored, cut in pieces, a small handful of fresh **spinach and kale,** 1 small **carrot**, peeled, cut in pieces, 1 small piece of **ginger**, peeled, a pinch of **turmeric,** 1 tsp **matcha** (green tea powder), 1 cup **orange juice**, juice of ¼ **lemon and zest.**

Tropical Green Shake

In a blender, combine until smooth:

1 cup **mango or papaya**, peeled and cut into chunks, ½ **banana**, peeled, ½ **apple**, cored and cut into chunks, 1½ cups fresh **spinach** leaves, 1 tsp each **flaxseeds and chia seeds,** ⅛ tsp **chlorella** powder, 1 cup **water** + 1 cup **coconut water** (or 2 cups of water only), ½ tsp **vanilla extract.** Optional: 1 tbsp of a **superfood powder**: lucuma, maca.

Complete Breakfast Smoothie

Inspired by JJ Virgin's smoothie blend (from her book *The Virgin Diet*), this my version of the smoothie full of vitamins, antioxidants, protein and omega-3. I use a NutriBullet to blend. A regular blender works well, too.

Blend all ingredients until smooth. Consume shortly after.

One big handful of a combination of baby spinach
leaves, mint leaves, parsley, various lettuce leaves
One handful of berries or ½ apple
One scoop of plant **protein powder**☺
2 tbsp of seeds and nuts of your choice
such as sesame, hemp, chia, flax, almonds,
pine nuts, walnuts, macadamia, etc.

Zest of an orange
Pinch of cinnamon
1 cup of coconut milk or coconut water
½ cup water

Banana Carrot Chai Smoothie

Sounds weird?
This deliciously soothing and nourishing smoothie has protein and fiber!
You will love this quick energizing drink to go.
No carrot juice? Use more almond or coconut milk and it will turn into a creamy banana chai.
Instead of reaching for a cup of coffee or a chocolate bar, this smoothie can make a
satisfying and healthy tie-me-over-dinner snack in the middle of the afternoon.

1 banana
½ cup almond milk or **coconut milk**☺
½ cup carrot juice
¼ tsp each ground cinnamon, cloves,
ginger, nutmeg and cardamom

1 tsp vanilla extract
Pinch of Celtic salt
1 scoop of **protein powder**☺
1 tbsp hemp seeds, flaxseeds or chia
seeds (or a combination of seeds)

Blend all ingredients in a blender. I like to use a NutriBullet for the smooth consistency that it gives to the drinks.

☺My favourite milk: **Organic Unsweetened Coconut Milk Beverage** from *So Delicious* for its taste and its short list of ingredients. My favourite **protein powder** is a blend from Vega containing plant protein, fiber and omega-3 blend; it is dairy-, gluten- and soy-free.

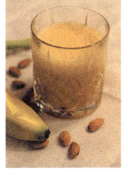

Spiced Apple Cider

Makes 6-8 cups
Prep Time: 10 min.
Warming Up Time: 20-30 min.

Philip often requests this autumn beverage, especially on a cold weekend afternoon when we just feel like cocooning at home. It doesn't seem to taste the same if I make it before October and after Christmas!

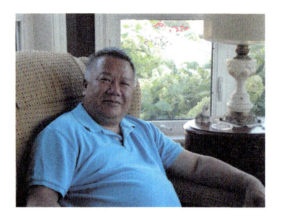

6-8 cups of apple cider
1 apple, cored and quartered
1 orange, unpeeled and quartered
1-2 cinnamon sticks
A handful of whole cloves

2 star anise
A 1-inch piece of fresh gingerroot, peeled
A handful of cardamom seeds
A handful of coriander seeds

1. In a large pot, warm up the apple cider on medium-low heat.
2. Add the apple pieces, and the orange quarters after squeezing them to release their juice.
3. Add the spices. Allow to become very fragrant and mouth-watering, about 20-30 minutes. If it is about to boil, turn the heat down.
4. Ladle into large mugs covered with a strainer to catch the spices. Return the spices to the pot. Serve and enjoy this very comforting cold-weather drink with your sweetie(s).

*"In the arithmetic of love, one plus one equals everything,
and two minus one equals nothing."*
-Mignon McLaughlin, U.S. journalist, playwright

Spanish Hot Chocolate

Makes 2 large mugs
Prep Time: 10 min.
Cooking Time: 10 min.

Here is a decadent but healthy occasional treat, and a must for Valentine's Day!

I love this beverage especially after coming back home from a cold winter outing, like "winter landscaping" (snow shoveling following a heavy snow fall). I look at it as my reward for having survived the strenuous activity, and my therapeutic remedy for sore muscles.

A hot mug of cocoa on a cold wintery day reminds me of my childhood: after school spending hours making snow forts with my brother, classmates and neighbours until my mother calling us to come in for dinner, a steaming hot chocolate waiting for us. Red cheeks and cold fingers tingling, noses running, tousled hair sticking up with static… Aaah! Happy, carefree childhood days when all you had to do was play and get along with your playmates!

Dark chocolate is a superfood that contains disease-fighting antioxidants and magnesium. The following combination of spices and cocoa helps ward off a cold and warm the soul. It may lower blood pressure and cholesterol. The comforting spicy sweet aroma calms the heart while it stimulates the senses. These are good enough reasons for me to go make this treat right now and call my neighbour over!

A. ½ cup water
1¼ cups milk + ¼ cup half & half
2½ tbsp sweetener of your choice
3-4 whole cloves
A pinch of ground ginger
A pinch or two of crushed red pepper
1 cinnamon stick
4-5 cardamom pods

B. ¼ cup unsweetened cocoa
1 tsp vanilla

1. In a small saucepan, combine the **A** ingredients. Bring to a boil and remove from heat.
2. With a whisk, stir in the **B** ingredients. Strain into 2 large mugs and enjoy.

Variations:

- Substitute almond milk for the cow's milk and half & half.
- For a richer delight, instead of the cocoa, use ¼ cup of 70% dark chocolate, grated or cut in pieces, then melted in a double boiler☺.
- In a separate pot, heat the milk, sweetener and the spices. Strain the milk mixture before slowly stirring in the melted chocolate.
- For the ultimate decadence: top the hot beverage with… whipped cream! Sinful but sooooo good! (Hey, I earned it: I just shoveled the driveway!)

☺Cooking in a double boiler, or *bain-Marie*, means cooking in a dish (pot or bowl) that is partially immersed in hot water.

Whetting the Appetite

Appetizers

I could easily live on appetizers and *small* plates alone!
I think it is a unique and exciting way to eat and entertain.
After one of these experiences,
I feel quite satisfied and comfortable - because I didn't stuff myself,
happy - because I sampled and tasted a variety of special, delightful treats,
and inspired - because I want to look up the recipes of my favourite delicacies to try at home.

The small plate concept is the foundation of many European and Asian menus:
an assortment of small portions that express a harmony of flavours.
These dishes often display all the great themes of the given country's lifestyle:
simplicity, elegance, fresh ingredients, attention to detail, and a delight in miniatures.
The Italians have *antipasti,*
the French have *hors d'œuvre* and *canapés,*
the Chinese have *dim sum,*
the Spanish have *tapas,*
and Greece and many Middle Eastern countries have *mezze.*

When eating out, I am always drawn to the appetizer section of the menu and negotiate with Philip how we could make a succulent and satisfying meal with several small dishes without ordering too much food.

I love the tapas style of eating because I feel that it captures the essence of the Art of eating well:
a tasting menu of varied bite-sized morsels that invites sharing – often standing up –
with friends and family, engaging in stimulating conversations, from sunrise to sunset,
in a relaxed atmosphere of celebration.

Two or three tapas or appetizers are perfect to serve before dinner as starters. Add a few more little dishes and you have a light meal or a lazy lunch. I rarely drink alcohol because I don't like the taste of most alcoholic beverages and the effect they have on me; however, I like the concept of Happy Hour (just the food for me, thank you!), perhaps once a week, featuring enticing and flavourful small plates that have great visual appeal. I see it as an occasion to gather, connect, and bond while sharing amazing food – culinary, intellectual and spiritual.

Pâté de foies de poulet
(French Chicken Liver Pâté)

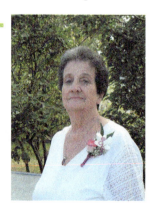

Makes 2 cups
Prep Time: 15 min.
Cooking Time: 1 hour
Chilling Time: a few hours to set in the refrigerator

My mother and I created this delicious and light pâté that can be served as an appetizer or enjoyed as a snack with apple pieces. You will notice that, unlike many pâtés, this one doesn't contain butter or cream.

¼ lb pancetta
2 garlic cloves, peeled
1 onion, peeled, quartered
1 shallot, quartered
½ lb chicken livers, cleaned and trimmed
1 tsp dried thyme

1 bay leaf
1 tsp dried savory or sage
A pinch of tarragon
A pinch of Celtic salt and black pepper
¾ cup water or chicken broth
2 tbsp Brandy (optional)

1. In a large frying pan, brown pancetta until almost crispy. Remove and set aside. Discard most of the oil, keeping enough to lightly cover the bottom of the pan.
2. Brown onion chunks, garlic cloves and shallot for a few minutes. Add livers, herbs, and seasonings. Cook for a few minutes until fragrant.
3. Add water or chicken broth and Brandy. Bring to a boil. Reduce heat and let simmer for 45 minutes, stirring occasionally.
4. Remove from heat and let cool to room temperature.
5. Purée in a food processor until a smooth consistency is achieved. After processing, for a smoother texture, press the mixture through a sieve over a bowl with a spatula. Discard the solid bits. Transfer to a serving bowl or ramekin, and refrigerate for a few hours to set. The texture is very soft and sets a little in the refrigerator.

Serving suggestions:

- Garnish with a sprig of fresh parsley, thyme or tarragon, and a few cracked pink peppercorns. Serve with sweet cornichons and pickled onions.
- It is very spreadable on crackers, cucumber slices and raw vegetables. It also makes a great filling for bite-size sandwiches.
- If you prefer a slightly coarser texture, you don't need to press the mixture through a sieve after processing.

Mousse au saumon
(Salmon Mousse)

Makes 2 cups
Prep Time: 15 min.
Cooking Time: 5 min.
Chilling Time: 3-4 hours in the refrigerator

You will like this versatile mousse. It disappears every time I serve it. Philip often requests it.

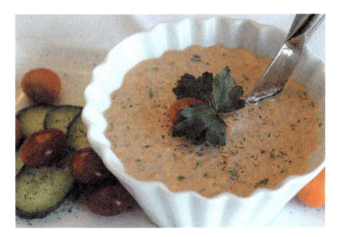

A- 1 envelope of unflavoured gelatin
¼ cup water

B- Seasoning: Mix in a bowl and set aside.
1 tbsp honey
1 tbsp lemon juice
2 tsp each of onion flakes and chives
½ tsp each of celery salt, celery seeds and chopped dill
¼ tsp each of paprika and cayenne pepper
The reserved juice from the salmon

C- 1 can salmon, (reserve the juice) boned, skinned and mashed with a fork
¾ cup celery, chopped
¼ cup each of mayonnaise and yogurt
1 tsp horseradish (optional, for a little kick)

1. In a small saucepan, sprinkle gelatin over water. Let stand 5 minutes. Over low heat, gently warm and stir to dissolve.
2. Add seasoning ingredients **(B)** and stir. Set aside.
3. In a mixing bowl, combine the **(C)** ingredients. Add the seasoning-gelatin mixture (**A** and **B**) and stir to combine.
4. Pour into a 2-cup mold or bowl. Cover with plastic wrap and chill well to set, about 3-4 hours.
5. Unmold (if desired), and decorate with cherry tomatoes and fresh herbs. Serve with crackers, lettuce leaves, and/or cucumber slices.

Variations:

- You can substitute canned tuna for the salmon, add chopped olives and chopped sun-dried tomatoes and chopped basil.
- You can add ¼ cup of chopped smoked salmon to the salmon mixture.
- You can omit step 1 (the gelatin) and use the mixture as a filling for sandwiches or lettuce wraps.

Spiced Nuts

Makes 2 cups
Prep Time: 5 min.
Cooking Time: 5 min.

You can use any nuts you like for this appetizer and snack. They all work well. You can adjust the quantity of the seasoning as well as the choice of spices to your liking. Instead of the five-spice, curry powder can be substituted.

¼ tsp Chinese five-spice
½ tsp or more chili powder
1 tsp cane sugar or sucanat or coconut sugar
1 tsp Celtic salt

2 cups of nuts such as almonds, cashews, pecans, walnuts, macadamia nuts
1 tsp (or more if needed) olive or vegetable oil

1. Preheat oven to 350°F.
2. Combine the spices, sugar and salt in a bowl and mix well.
3. Place the nuts onto a baking sheet. Using your hands or a spatula, coat the nuts with the oil. Sprinkle with the spice mix, toss to coat. Roast in the oven for 5 minutes until golden, stirring frequently to prevent burning.
4. Serve warm from the oven or at room temperature.

Sun-dried Tomato Tapenade

Makes 1½ cups
Prep Time: 10 min.

1 cup pitted black olives
2 garlic cloves, minced
3 anchovy fillets, rinsed
3 tbsp capers, rinsed and drained
¼ tsp lemon zest

4 tbsp chopped fresh herbs such as cilantro, mint, parsley, basil
1½ tbsp lemon juice
Ground black pepper
½ cup oil-packed, sun-dried tomatoes
Oil from sun-dried tomatoes, olive oil

1. Place olives, garlic, anchovy fillets, capers, zest and herbs in a food processor. Blend until smooth.
2. Add lemon juice and pepper. Add enough oil from the sun-dried tomatoes to make a paste. Add sun-dried tomatoes and blend for 20 seconds.
3. Serve with toasted **Bread** slices from the **Wholesome and Nourishing Baking** section or **Crackers**.
4. You can also serve it in hollowed cherry tomatoes, on cucumber rounds, or in endive leaves.

French Chicken and Vegetable Galantine

Serves 6-8
Prep Time: 30 min.
Cooking Time: 20 min.
Chilling Time: several hours

If you need a dish that is colourful, pretty and tasty for a brunch or buffet meal,
this Galantine is a great item to include in your menu. It can be prepared the day before.

1 tbsp each of olive oil and butter
1 onion, chopped
½ red pepper, chopped
½ green pepper, chopped
1 celery stalk, chopped
6-8 mushrooms, chopped
1-2 cooked organic chicken or turkey breast(s), boneless and skinless

¼ lb pancetta or bacon, cooked until crispy
1-2 envelope(s) unflavoured gelatin
Chicken broth
Celtic salt and pepper
Fresh parsley, thyme, basil and oregano, chopped
A good pinch of paprika and sage

1. Melt the butter and the oil in a frying pan. Sauté onion, peppers, celery, mushrooms and fresh herbs until fragrant. Let cool.
2. Cut the cooked chicken or turkey into small pieces. Place in a large bowl. Add the vegetable mixture to chicken.
3. Cut pancetta in small pieces. Add to chicken-vegetable mixture. Mix together.
4. In a small saucepan, sprinkle the gelatin in ¼ cup water and allow to soften for 5 minutes. Gently stir over medium-low heat to dissolve.
5. Add chicken broth, salt, pepper, herbs and paprika to the dissolved gelatin. Stir to combine.
6. Pour the gelatin mixture in the chicken-vegetable bowl, and stir. Transfer into a 6-8 cup mould. Refrigerate for several hours.
7. To serve, spoon individual portions out or cut into triangular wedges.

Variations:

- Add sun-dried tomatoes to the vegetable mix.
- Replace the fresh red pepper with roasted red peppers.
- You can use a variety of mushrooms i.e., oyster, cremini.
- You can serve it in small spoons or tiny clear glasses as individual appetizers.
- With a green salad, a slice of this galantine makes a delicious and light spa lunch.

"The first wealth is health."
--Ralph Waldo Emerson

Mediter-asian Cocktail Skewers

Serves 4-6
Prep Time: 40-50 min.

These classy, no-cook appetizers are easy to prepare and will please any crowd. Depending on the amount of supplies that you have, you could make 4 to 6 of each skewer type, so your guests could sample all of them. I like to use short metal or bamboo skewers. I arrange the cocktail skewers on a large platter for great visual and gustatory appeal. I always bring the empty platter back to the kitchen!

On each skewer, thread the following ingredients:

Italian Classic: cubes of mozzarella wrapped with ½ slice of prosciutto, and cantaloupe cubes or balls carved with a melon baller. Sprinkle each skewer with black pepper and chopped fresh rosemary or basil. Drizzle with some extra-virgin olive oil and a little balsamic vinegar.

Italian Caprese: cherry tomatoes, bocconcini balls (1" in diameter), fresh basil leaves. Season with Celtic salt and pepper. Drizzle some extra-virgin olive oil and a little balsamic vinegar.

Italian Pesto Treat: in a Ziploc plastic bag, combine cherry tomatoes, salami slices cut into half-moons, pieces of red pepper, black olives, and 1-2 tbsp pesto (store-bought or home-made). Close the bag and gently massage the contents to evenly coat them with the pesto. Thread the skewers with the pesto-covered ingredients and a fresh basil leaf.

Niçoise: ¼ hard-cooked egg, a cherry tomato, an olive, a basil leaf, a cooked snow pea or green bean cut in half. Drizzle with some olive oil and sprinkle with Celtic salt and cracked black pepper.

Greek 1: a cooked shrimp, an olive, a cube of feta cheese, a cherry tomato, a small piece of green pepper. Sprinkle with finely chopped fresh oregano, Celtic salt and pepper. Drizzle with olive oil.

Greek 2: a blue or red seedless grape, a cube of firm feta, 1 small fresh mint leaf (if the leaf is too large, cut it in half). Drizzle over the skewers 1 tbsp liquid honey, and sprinkle some fennel seeds and finely chopped mint leaves.

Spanish: a slice of chorizo, a small piece of red pepper, a cube of manchego cheese, an olive. Drizzle with olive oil. Sprinkle with a little hot pepper flakes and some finely chopped parsley or coriander.

Thai: a piece of cooked chicken, a slice of mango, a small piece of red pepper, a fresh basil leaf. Sprinkle with some lime zest. In a small bowl, combine a little tamari, lime juice, grated ginger, a little bit of liquid honey, and some finely chopped coriander. Drizzle over the skewers.

Asian Rainbow: a lychee, a cube of pineapple, a piece of mango, a cube of watermelon, and a blue grape. Drizzle with a little bit of liquid honey and lime juice. Sprinkle some lime zest, black sesame seeds, and finely cut mint leaves.

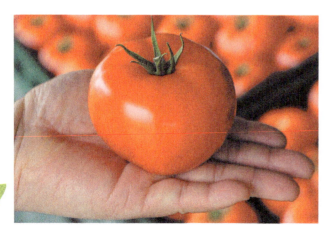
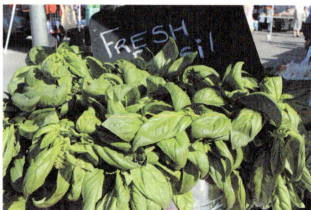

Crevettes et légumes avec leur sauce verte
(Shrimp and Vegetables with a Green Sauce)

Serves 6-8
Prep Time: 30 min.
Cooking Time: 30 min.

Quite attractive and sustaining, this appetizer consisting of a colourful assortment of fresh and cooked "dippers" can also be served as a light lunch for 2-4 people. It is an ideal menu to enjoy when the fresh summer produce are at their peak of perfection. The water used to cook the vegetables and the shrimp is quite flavourful to drink or reserved for a soup.

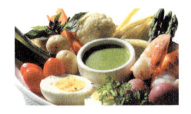

Sauce verte:

1 garlic clove
1 cup olive oil
¼ cup white wine vinegar
2 tbsp Dijon mustard
1 tsp lemon zest
1 tsp orange zest

½ cup of a combination of chopped fresh herb: parsley, coriander, mint, basil, chives
¼ cup spinach leaves, chopped
¼ tsp paprika or hot red pepper flakes or *piment d'Espelette*
Celtic salt and pepper

Platter:

¾ lb large red potatoes, or small potatoes, or fingerlings
Celtic salt and pepper
¾ lb carrots, cut into sticks, or whole young carrots
¾ lb cauliflower, cut in florets
¾ lb asparagus, trimmed
¾ lb green and yellow beans, ends trimmed

¾ lb large shrimp, shelled, deveined
4 hard-boiled eggs, shelled, quartered
1-2 zucchinis, cut in half, then into sticks; they can be steamed or kept raw
2 cup cherry tomatoes
Chopped parsley

Sauce verte:

1. In a blender, place the garlic, the oil and the vinegar. Blend until smooth and thick.
2. Add the rest of the ingredients. Blend until smooth. Divide among 4 non-metallic dipping bowls, if serving as individual appetizers.

Platter:

1. In a large saucepan, cover potatoes with salted water. Bring to a boil; then, simmer. Cook partially covered until fork-tender, 20-25 minutes. Drain and transfer to a large serving platter; quarter if using large potatoes.
2. In the meantime, in a medium saucepan, cover carrots with water; add a bit of salt. Bring to a boil; then, simmer. Cook until tender, about 5 minutes. Drain and transfer to the serving platter.
3. Cook cauliflower, asparagus, and beans in the water until tender, 6-8 minutes. Drain and transfer to the serving platter.
4. Cook shrimp in the water until pink, 1-2 minutes. Drain and transfer to the serving platter.
5. Arrange the potatoes, the eggs, the shrimp and the vegetables attractively on the large platter, or on individual small appetizer plates. Sprinkle with parsley. Serve warm with the **sauce verte.**

Warming the Soul

Soups

Are you one of those people who must start a meal with a soup because a meal is not complete without one?
You are in good company!

In my opinion, every day is a soup day, regardless of the weather and the temperature outside.
A hot vegetable soup (with or without protein) makes a great light lunch. If I am
still hungry, a salad or some cooked vegetables round off the meal. Most soups taste
even better the next day, making them a leftover I look forward to.
They are easy to warm up and pack in a thermos for lunch or a snack on the go.
I think they are the best and healthiest *fast food!*

Soups are very versatile. All you need is some inspiration, -- which is often provided by hunger --
and a few basic ingredients on hand. You can put pretty much anything in them:
water, broth, juices, wine, coconut milk, vegetables, fruits, meat, seafood, spices, herbs,
egg crêpe cut thinly like noodles, eggs, Paleo breads, crackers, and *croûtons*.
(Even a stone! Remember the children's story about the stone soup?)
Vary the ingredients and you have a whole new experience every time.

Some soups can be prepared quickly while others need more simmering time to build flavour.
Their texture can be chunky, creamy-velvety, half chunky-half creamy, or clear.

A simple homemade clear vegetable-base broth is often what I choose to ingest
when I am not feeling well as it seems to nourish, rebalance
and get me back to my old self more quickly.

So, come on over! The soup's on!

Italian Stracciatella

Serves 6
Prep Time: 5-10 min.
Cooking Time: 10-15 min.

This light Italian soup is so easy and quick to make.
It is perfect for when you are in a hurry and you only
have these basic ingredients in your refrigerator.
You can omit the cheese, if necessary.

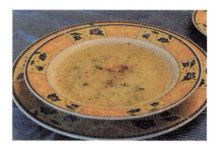

8 cups organic chicken broth
2 eggs
½ cup grated Parmigiano-Reggiano (optional)
2 tbsp chopped Italian parsley

Lemon juice
Celtic salt and pepper
Pinch of ground hot red pepper (optional)

1. Bring the chicken broth to a boil over medium-high heat. Reduce the heat to medium-low and simmer.
2. Beat the eggs in a mixing bowl, and add the cheese and parsley.
3. Slowly pour the egg mixture into the broth, stirring with a whisk. The faster you stir, the finer the pieces of egg --the eggs take on the appearance of *straccetti* or little rags.
4. Season to taste with lemon juice, salt, pepper and hot pepper, if desired.

Thai Scallops and Spinach Soup

Serves 4
Prep Time: 10 min.
Cooking Time: 15-20 min.

I love the colours of this soup: white, bright green and little specks of red.
No scallops? Substitute with the same amount of shrimp. Or use chicken pieces.

A- 1½ cups chicken broth
1 tbsp lemongrass, cut finely
2 green onions, chopped
½ red chili, seeded and finely chopped
½ green bell pepper, seeded and finely chopped
A handful of enoki mushrooms (or
white mushrooms, thinly sliced)
½ tsp cane sugar or maple syrup
1 tbsp fish sauce
Juice of 1 lime

B- 2 tbsp vegetable oil
6-8 scallops, rinsed and patted dry, each
one sliced horizontally in 2 thin disks
2 large handfuls of fresh spinach leaves

1. In a saucepan, put all the ingredients from the **A** section, and simmer for 8-10 minutes.
2. In a heavy skillet, heat the oil on high heat. When hot, sear the scallops for about 1 minute on each side until just cooked and lightly golden, so they don't become tough.
3. Add the spinach to the broth and continue to simmer until the leaves have just wilted, about a minute. Taste the broth and adjust the seasoning, if needed. Serve the soup in bowls and add the scallops on top.

Spanish Gazpacho

Serves 6-8
Prep Time: 30 min.
Cooling Time: several hours
Standing Time: 1½ hours

This no-cook soup should be made 1 day ahead to allow the flavours to marry.
You will find that this is a refreshing and colourful soup, perfect for a hot summer day gathering.
Your guests will be impressed. Olé!

A. 1 garlic clove, crushed
¼ sweet onion, minced
½ green pepper, and ½ red pepper, minced
2 large tomatoes, peeled, seeded, thinly minced
½ English cucumber, peeled, seeded and thinly minced
1 celery, threads removed, minced
1 jalapeño pepper, seeded and minced
⅛ of a ripe Cranshaw or honeydew
melon, minced. Reserve its juice.
Any juicy fruits: mango, papaya, melon, thinly chopped
1 box of vegetable juice

B. Seasoning:
Salt and pepper
Juice of ½ lemon
1 tbsp vinegar or sherry vinegar
2 blood oranges, zested and juiced
2 tbsp tarragon oil☺
¼ cup parsley and coriander, finely chopped for garnish

1. In a stainless steel bowl, combine the **A** ingredients. Mix well.
2. Refrigerate for several hours, preferably overnight.
3. In a food processor, blend half of the mixture. Return to the coarse mixture and mix well.
4. Add the **B** ingredients and allow the gazpacho to stand at room temperature for 1½ hours.
5. Serve in individual cups, garnished with parsley and coriander. Serve with crackers or gluten-free toasts.

☺ Tarragon oil: In a saucepan, warm ¼ cup of olive oil with a few leaves of fresh tarragon until they become a little crispy.

Variations:

- You can purée the whole gazpacho in a blender, and pour it in an ice cream maker to be served as a sorbet.
- You could use only fruits and serve the gazpacho as a cool summer dessert.

My favourite delicious movies and books:

Vatel
Waitress
Chocolat
Ratatouille
Just Desserts
Julie & Julia
No Reservations
Like Water for Chocolate
The Hundred-foot Journey

Crème de citrouille
(Cream of Pumpkin)

Serves 2-4
Prep Time: 15 min.
Cooking Time: 25 min.

To save some time, instead of peeling and cooking the whole pumpkin, I use a can of organic pumpkin flesh. This is a warming and comforting soup for the cold months.

1 tbsp olive or coconut oil
1 onion, finely chopped
1 carrot, finely chopped
1 celery stalk, chopped
1 bay leaf
1 15-oz can of organic pumpkin flesh
¼ tsp ground clove

1 tsp aniseeds
Celtic salt and pepper
3 cups of water or chicken broth
A pinch of saffron
Fresh parsley to garnish
Bacon slices, cooked until crispy

1. Heat the oil in a saucepan over medium-low heat. Add the onion, carrot, celery, and bay leaf. Cook for a few minutes until softened and fragrant.
2. Stir in the pumpkin flesh, clove, aniseeds, salt and pepper. Pour in the water or broth. Add the saffron.
3. Bring to a boil; then, lower the heat and simmer gently for 15-20 minutes.
4. If you want the soup to be very creamy, you can blend it to the desired consistency.
5. Serve hot, sprinkled with parsley, and accompanied with bacon slices that you dip in the soup. Or break the bacon slices in pieces that you sprinkle on top of the soup.

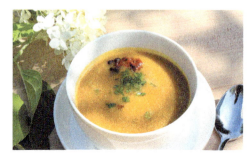

Chinese Wrapper-less Wonton Soup

Serves 4
Prep Time: 30-45 min.
Cooking Time: 30-35 min.

This "paleotized" version can be made with a variety of ground meat from chicken and pork to chopped shrimp. The beaten egg should help keep the mixture together; however, it is possible that the meat balls fall apart in the soup. It is quite all right, it adds great flavour to the broth.

Broth:
4 cups chicken broth, organic or homemade
1 carrot, peeled and grated
1 celery stalk, cut in chunks
1 onion, quartered
1 piece of ginger of about 1 inch

Soup:
1 tbsp organic tamari
1 tbsp rice wine
½ tsp sesame oil
1 head of baby bok choy, thinly sliced
3-4 white mushrooms, sliced
To garnish: 1 thinly sliced green onion, and 2 tbsp of chopped coriander

Wonton:
½ lb ground turkey or veal
2 tbsp water chestnut, finely chopped (You can find them in cans in Asian food markets.)
½ tsp hot pepper flakes
1 tbsp coriander, finely chopped
1 tsp organic tamari
1 tsp sesame oil
½ tsp ground black pepper
1 egg, lightly beaten

1. In a stockpot or large saucepan, bring the **broth** ingredients to a boil. Turn heat down and allow to simmer for 10-15 minutes to develop flavour.
2. While the broth is simmering, prepare the **wontons**. In a mixing bowl, combine the **wonton** ingredients together. Using a teaspoon as a guide, gather some of the meat mixture to form balls. Add the meat balls to the broth and cook for a few minutes.
3. Add the **soup** ingredients except the green onion and coriander. Simmer gently for 10 minutes.
4. Ladle the soup into bowls and garnish with the green onions and the coriander.

It is my understanding that
God gives us three answers to our prayers:
"Yes!"
"Not yet!"
"I have something better for you!"

Thai Butternut Squash and Shrimp Curry

Serves 4
Prep Time: ½ hour
Cooking Time of Stock: ½ hour
Cooking Time of Soup: ½ hour

I love a mildly spicy curry! If you don't, you can omit the red chili pepper and add only a pinch of red pepper flakes. If you don't want to make the simple seafood stock, you can use water or even chicken broth. You can serve this versatile and fragrant stew-like dish as a soup with chicken or beef strips instead that you brown first, or allow to cook in chicken broth or water in step 4.

2 shallots, sliced	1 can of coconut milk
2 tbsp coconut oil	1½ cups of seafood stock☺
1 garlic clove, chopped	1 tsp fish sauce
1 tsp gingerroot, grated	1 tsp of palm sugar or coconut sugar
1 fresh red chili pepper, seeded and sliced	1 lime, zested and juiced
1 lemongrass stem, crushed and cut into 2-inch pieces	1 lb raw shrimp, shelled (reserve the shells
2 tsp ground turmeric	for the seafood stock) and deveined
1 tsp ground coriander	Fresh coriander to garnish
½-1 lb butternut squash, peeled and cut into 1-inch cubes	

☺**Simple Seafood Stock:**

In a saucepan, place the **shrimp shells**, and cover with water. Add 1 tsp of salt and bring to a boil. Skim and discard the foam. Add **1-2 carrots**, peeled and cut in a few pieces, **1 onion**, peeled and cut into quarters, **1-2 celery sticks**, cut in a few pieces. Bring the stock back to boiling. Remove any foam from the surface and lower the heat. Cook until the carrots are tender. Strain the liquid and reserve. You can discard the solids as they have served their purpose.

1. In a saucepan, gently fry the shallots in the oil for a few minutes. Add the garlic, ginger, chili, lemongrass and spices, and cook for 1 minute or so.
2. Add the butternut squash and stir to coat with the spices.
3. Gradually stir in the coconut milk, seafood stock, fish sauce, sugar and lime zest. Bring to a boil; then, lower the heat and simmer for 15 minutes or so.
4. Add the shrimp and cook for 4-5 minutes. Stir in the lime juice.
5. Serve in bowls and garnish with coriander.

Vichyssoise
(French Leeks Soup)

Serves 6
Prep Time: 10 min.
Cooking Time: 20-30 min.

This easy and simple soup is from my mother.
You can serve it as thick as you like.

3-4 leeks, white and light green parts only	1 celery stalk, chopped
1 tbsp olive or butter oil	Celtic salt and pepper
2 medium potatoes, peeled and chopped in small cubes	4-6 cups of water or chicken broth for a richer flavour

1. Slice the leeks in half, lengthwise. Rinse well between the layers to remove all sand and dirt. Chop crosswise in thin half-moon slices.
2. Heat the oil in a pot over medium heat. Add the leeks and gently cook for a few minutes. Do not allow to brown or burn. Add the potatoes and celery, and cook for a few minutes. Season with salt and pepper.
3. Add water or broth and bring to a boil. Simmer until very tender and fragrant. Check the seasoning.
4. Here are a few serving options:

   - enjoy it chunky as it is,
   - mash it with a potato masher,
   - purée the soup and enjoy it creamy,
   - purée and strain it for a liquid consistency,
   - eat the soup while it is still warm, or chill it before serving,
   - garnish with finely chopped chives and grated parmesan.

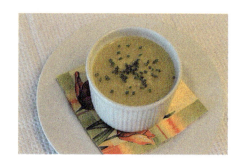

Simple Chicken Soup

Serves 4-6
Prep Time: 20 min.
Cooking Time: 20 min.

This simple and wonderful soup derives from the leftover meat and broth created in the **No-fuss Chicken Dinner** found in the **Flying Protein (Chicken)** section. I used to add short pasta or egg noodles. I occasionally top the soup with **Egg Crêpes** cut in ½-inch strips. Please refer to the **Starting the Day (Breakfast)** section for the **Egg Crêpes** recipe.

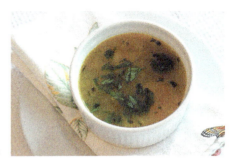

This soup does wonders when it feels like you are coming down with a cold. Its pungent and spicy ingredients have been a favoured treatment for colds and other respiratory concerns for centuries. The salty liquid soothes a sore throat and helps rehydrate the body if there is a fever. The chunks of meat and vegetables provide health-giving nutrients you might not ingest if your appetite is diminished. And if you generously add onions, garlic and spices in the soup, you may experience relief from nasal congestion, and possibly, some stirring up and ejection of phlegm in the bronchial passageway. To be ready in the event that you or someone in your household comes down with a cold, you may want to freeze containers of your homemade stock and soups early in the cold season.

1 tsp each of butter and olive oil
1 sweet onion, peeled, diced
2 carrots, peeled, diced
2 celery stalks, diced
1 tsp or more curry powder
Pinch of Celtic salt

Black pepper
4 cups chicken broth, including the cooking liquid from the **No-fuss Chicken Dinner** recipe
2-3 cups of cooked chicken meat, cut into small cubes
Egg Crêpes, if using
2 tbsp fresh parsley, finely chopped, for garnish

1. In a saucepan, heat the butter and oil over medium heat.
2. Add the onion and cook for a few minutes until softened. Add the carrots and celery. Cook for 3-5 minutes. Sprinkle the curry powder, salt and pepper; stir to coat until fragrant, about 1-2 minutes.
3. Pour in the broth (and gelatin from the **No-fuss Chicken Dinner**). Bring to a boil; reduce to a simmer. Cook until the carrots are tender.
4. Add the cooked chicken cubes, and the egg crêpe strips; stir to heat through. Taste and adjust the seasoning, if needed.
5. Ladle into soup bowls, garnish with parsley.

Chicken Stock

(Makes 10-12 cups)

In many of my recipes, I use chicken stock for its flavour and nutrients. When I make a large batch of broth or stock, I freeze what I won't use immediately in 2-cup Ziploc containers, label and date. It keeps up to 4 months in the freezer. To thaw, I run some hot tap water around the outside of the plastic container to dislodge the frozen stock. Once it is dislodged from the sides of the container, the frozen mass can be transferred to a saucepan. Over low heat, I let it gradually melt and liquefy. I love drinking this stock warm with some chopped chives as garnish. It is filling and comforting.

3-5 lbs of chicken parts (legs, wings, necks, gizzards, and/or bones; whatever you can find. It all gives great flavour.)
2-3 onions, peeled and quartered
4-6 carrots, peeled, cut in halves
3-5 celery stalks with leaves, cut in halves

2 parsnips, peeled, cut in halves
1 garlic clove, peeled, cut in half
Large handfuls of fresh herbs like parsley, dill, thyme
2 bay leaves
1-2 tbsp Celtic salt
1 tsp whole black peppercorns

Place the chicken parts in a large stockpot with enough water to cover the contents and one or two inches above. Bring to a boil. With a slotted spoon, skim the foam that comes up to the surface. Once there is no more foam to skim, add the rest of the ingredients. Bring to a boil again. Turn the heat down and simmer, uncovered, for 2-3 hours. If you are hungry and anxious to have a taste of this wonderfully fragrant nectar, you may eat the chicken and vegetables with a little broth as a soup. Strain the rest of the liquid in a colander or a sieve. Discard the herbs. Chill. When chilled, the coagulated fat can be removed from the surface with a spoon, and discarded. Pour into containers, label and date before freezing.

Vegetable Stock

(Makes 8 cups)

This vitamin-rich broth can be used as:

- a base for a hearty vegetable soup,
- extra flavouring to a vegetable braise,
- a substitute for chicken stock in a soup,
- a warm beverage to give to someone who is not feeling well,
- part of a cleanse when cutting down on food intake is needed, and when it is time to do an internal spring cleaning.

2 onions, peeled, quartered	4 tomatoes, seeded and quartered
4 celery stalks with leaves, cut in chunks	1 garlic clove, peeled
4 carrots, peeled, cut in chunks	6-8 mushrooms, stemmed, cut in halves
1 parsnip, peeled, cut in chunks	Handfuls of fresh herbs like parsley, coriander, basil
1 leek, white part only, cleaned, cut in chunks	1 sprig of fresh dill
1 zucchini, trimmed, cut in thick slices	2 bay leaves
1 red pepper, stemmed, seeded, cut in chunks	10 black peppercorns
1 green pepper, stemmed, seeded, cut in chunks	½ tsp hot pepper flakes

Put all ingredients in a large stockpot. Bring to a boil; lower the heat, and simmer, uncovered for 2 hours. Strain the stock; discard the solids. Let cool to room temperature. Pour in storage containers, label and date. Freeze what you won't be using in the next few days.

Fish or Seafood Stock

(Makes 3-4 cups)

To add great flavour to the stock, you can use any seafood shell (crab, lobster, shrimp) saved from a previous meal, as well as fish heads. In a large stockpot, place the **shells and/or fish heads**. Add **water** and **½ cup of wine**, and bring to a boil. Skim the foam that comes to the surface. Add **1 carrot**, peeled and cut in chunks, **1 celery stalk**, cut in chunks, **1 onion**, peeled and cut in quarters, **Celtic salt** and **pepper**. Bring to a boil again; then, reduce the heat. Add **a handful of parsley sprigs** and simmer for 20 minutes. Strain the liquid and reserve. If you like, you can eat the tasty vegetables and the meat in the fish heads. Otherwise, they can be discarded. The excess stock can be frozen in 2-cup Ziploc plastic containers for future use. Remember to label and date the containers.

Loading Up on the Greens

Salads and Vegetable Dishes

My favourite section of any cookbook! (Other than the fruit desserts section, of course!) Raw from the garden, steamed, sautéed, braised, boiled, grilled, roasted; they are all so *good*! They are the foundation of the spa cuisine.

At every meal (fine, most meals!), I aim at filling 75-85% of my plate or bowl with a variety of vegetables, raw and cooked. It allows me to fill up with what my body thrives on while leaving little room for what I shouldn't eat on a regular basis.

After years of discomfort and low energy, I finally figured out what works for me and it wouldn't be wise on my part to not respect that. The body that the Creator gave me is the only vehicle I have in this life with which to live my passions and dreams, and to accomplish my mission of being of service to others. In appreciation for this wonderfully well-functioning body, I want to treat it with respect, and honor its nature by providing it with loving care and the best nourishment.

I see good-quality nourishment as daily investments toward my long-term immunity, comfort, and longevity. Nothing can imitate products from Mother Nature and claim to be as good, tasty, effective and healing. No one can convince me that processed food (nutrient-deficient and toxic to the body) and synthetic drugs are better than the food and remedies from Mother Nature. We are creatures of Nature; it makes sense that what keeps us alive and well comes from Nature. For this reason, I have purposefully created longer chapters focusing on produce, like this one, with more than 20 vegetable recipes.

So, feel comfortable to eat large quantities of raw and cooked vegetables for lunch and dinner, and even breakfast! They are Nature's remedy for many health issues as they are filled with phytonutrients, antioxidants, fiber, vitamins, minerals, proteins, and water -- all essential elements to reach and maintain vibrant health and longevity. Remember, when you fill up on plant food, there isn't much room for unhealthy foods that create cravings, addictions and overeating.
A bonus: vegetables are naturally **hypo-caloric**!

Shredded Carrots with Toasted Almonds

Serves 4
Prep Time: 10 min.

This is a quick salad made with simple ingredients that most likely you would have on hand. The children like its sweet crunchiness.

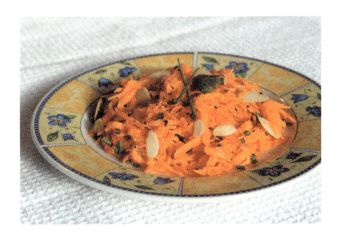

Dressing:
5-6 tbsp flaxseed oil (or olive oil)
1 tsp lemon juice
1 tbsp orange juice
1 tsp orange zest
1 tbsp orange marmalade
1½ tsp horseradish

Salad:
1 lb carrots, shredded or grated
½ cup sliced almonds, toasted
1 tbsp chopped chives
Celtic salt and pepper

1. **Dressing:** In a screw-top glass jar, combine the ingredients. Screw the lid on and shake vigorously until creamy and emulsified.
2. In a large bowl, combine carrots and almonds. Add some of the dressing and toss until well coated, adding more if necessary. Taste the seasoning and adjust it if needed. Garnish with chives and season with salt and pepper.

Moroccan Roasted Red Peppers Salad

Serves 4
Prep Time: 20 min.
Roasting Time: 20-25 min.

This colourful and attractive salad can be served as a starter or a side dish to grilled meats.
Use peppers of different colours or just one variety.

3 plump bell peppers, red, orange or yellow,
a combination of various colours
2 tbsp olive oil
½ cup of parmesan chunks (optional)
¼ of a red onion or a handful of chopped chives

A handful of fresh parsley, finely chopped
Rind of ½ preserved lemon, cut in
thin slices, or orange zest
½ cup fresh green olives

1. Preheat the broiler or the barbecue.
2. Put the peppers on a baking dish; drizzle the oil over them. Put them in the oven or on the grill and roast them, turning them over often to allow the flesh to evenly soften, the skin to evenly char and wrinkle.
3. Remove the baking dish from the oven. Transfer the roasted peppers to a paper bag (or place them in a bowl; then, cover with plastic wrap) and let them soften and cool for a few minutes. Reserve any leftover roasting oil from the dish. When cooled, remove the pepper stems, scrape the seeds and peel the skins.
4. Slice lengthwise each pepper in quarters and place on a serving dish.
5. Arrange the parmesan chunks over the peppers. Scatter the chopped onion or chives, and the parsley over the peppers. Drizzle the roasting oil over the peppers and scatter the preserved lemon slices or orange zest. Scatter the olives over the salad. Season with ground black pepper and Celtic salt if you are not using the preserved lemon. Serve while still warm. If desired, you can serve the salad on a bed of arugula and top it with toasted pine nuts.

Orange and Carrot Salad with Pancetta Crisps

Serves 4
Prep Time: 20-25 min.
Cooking Time: 5-8 min.

The unusual combination of ingredients in this colourful salad
creates exotic flavours and interesting textures that I am sure you will fall in love with.
I did!

Dressing:	**Salad:**

Dressing:
In a screw-top glass jar, combine the following ingredients. Screw the lid on and shake vigorously to combine. Taste and adjust the seasoning, if necessary.
1 tbsp lemon juice
2 tsp cane sugar or sucanat
¼ tsp Celtic salt
1 tbsp orange blossom water
Pinch of cinnamon

Salad:
12 pancetta slices
1 head of Bibb lettuce or romaine lettuce, torn in smaller pieces
2 carrots, finely grated
2 oranges, peeled, and cut into skinless segments (*suprêmes*)
½ cup dates, stoned and cut into thin strips
Chopped parsley
¼ cup almonds, toasted and coarsely chopped
Optional: a pinch or more of hot red pepper

1. In a frying pan, working in batches, crisp the pancetta slices over medium heat. Allow to cool and drain on paper towels.
2. Arrange the lettuce leaves on the bottom and the inner sides of a salad bowl, or on individual serving plates.
3. Arrange the carrots in a mound in the middle. Place the orange segments around the carrot mound. Scatter the dates on top. Sprinkle the parsley and the almonds. Add the hot pepper, if using.
4. Arrange the pancetta crisps "standing up" around the carrot-orange-date mound.
5. Drizzle some of the dressing and serve.

☺**Here is how to cut** *suprêmes* **from an orange:**

Cut both ends of the orange off. Cut the peel around the flesh, exposing the segments; then, over the salad bowl to collect the juices, carefully slice on either sides of each membrane and release the "naked" segments into the bowl. Keep the juice to add to a vinaigrette or a drink. Visit my website at www.olivestolychees.com for a demonstration.

Did you know that the medjool date is called the King of the dates?
That is because it is sweeter than the other common dates.

Japanese Avocado and Wakame Salad

Serves 4
Prep Time: 20-30 min.
Cooking Time: 10 min.

I was inspired by a colourful salad I once had at a Japanese restaurant. Here is my version of it.

Wakame is a kind of seaweed, rich in nutrients and trace minerals from the sea. You can find packages of dried seaweeds in many Asian markets, fish markets and health food stores. If the pieces are too big, you can cut them with scissors in one-inch pieces or smaller. Soak the pieces for a few minutes in cold water to soften and reconstitute them to their original shape. After you have drained and squeezed them well in a towel, you can toss them in the salad bowl with the other ingredients.

Salad:

½ cup dried wakame that has been soaked for a few minutes in cold water and well drained (or use a combination of other seaweeds such as arame, dulse, kelp)
4 cups of washed, roughly chopped lettuce leaves
1 avocado, pitted and cut in long slices

½ cucumber, seeded and cut in half-moons
1 carrot, peeled, cut in half and julienned
A handful of sweet cherry tomatoes, cut in half
4 shrimp, shelled, deveined and cooked (baked, pan-fried or grilled)
2 tbsp sesame seeds

Option 1- Carrot-Ginger Dressing:

2 medium carrots, peeled
1 small shallot, roughly chopped
1 2-inch piece of gingerroot, peeled and roughly chopped
1-2 tbsp almond butter☺

1-2 tbsp rice vinegar
¼ cup water
2-3 tbsp vegetable oil
2 tbsp sesame oil

Option 2- Ginger-Tahini Dressing:

3 tbsp tahini☺
1 tsp grated gingerroot
2 tbsp lemon juice
1 tbsp sesame seed oil

1 tbsp non-GMO organic white miso
1 grated carrot
1 tbsp maple syrup
½ - ¾ cup water

Dressing (both options):

In a food processor or blender, process all ingredients of either option until well combined, and you can see only little bits of carrots. Taste and adjust the seasoning to your palate. Transfer to a screw-top glass jar and keep refrigerated until serving time. It will keep for 1 week refrigerated.

Salad:

In 4 salad plates, divide the lettuce leaves, the wakame, the avocado slices, the cucumber half-moons, the carrot strips and the tomato halves. Top with a shrimp and sesame seeds. Drizzle generously the dressing over. Your guests will love it!

☺Instead of the almond butter, I like to use a non-GMO organic white miso that can be purchased in Asian markets or health food stores. Tahini is a sesame seed paste sold in jars. You can find it in most grocery stores.

Mandarin Orange Almond Salad

Serves 4-6
Prep Time: 10-15 min.

I found the inspiration for this recipe from a salad I once had at a restaurant in Toulon, France. It is the mandarin oranges that make this salad so refreshing and interesting.

1 large head of romaine lettuce or
a variety of salad greens
1 cup chopped celery
2 tbsp finely chopped parsley

1 handful of chives, finely cut with scissors
1 10-oz can of mandarin oranges, drained
¼ cup toasted sliced almonds

Salad: Wash and dry lettuce, removing all the water from the leaves. When ready to serve, tear into bite-size pieces. Add celery, parsley, chives and mandarin oranges, and toss. To serve, sprinkle with the almonds and drizzle some of the vinaigrette over the salad.

Vinaigrette: Put the following ingredients in a screw-top glass jar. Screw the lid on and shake vigorously to combine, emulsify until it turns creamy white. Set aside.

1 tsp dried tarragon leaves
½ tsp each Celtic salt and pepper
1 tbsp sucanat or coconut sugar

½ tsp Dijon mustard
2-3 tbsp white wine vinegar
2-3 tbsp light olive oil

The Five 'C' Salad

Serves 2
Prep Time: 10-15 min.

The vibrant green colour of the herbs against the lively orange of the carrots makes this salad very appetizing and full of antioxidants. For an extra splash of bright colour, you can add purple and/or yellow carrots, if you happen to find some.

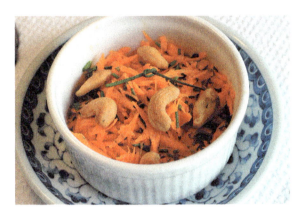

Dressing:
2 tbsp lemon or orange juice
2 tsp lemon or orange zest
½ tsp **C**umin or **C**araway seeds
2-3 tbsp olive oil
Celtic salt and pepper

Salad:
2-3 medium **C**arrots, shredded
3 sprigs of fresh **C**oriander, chopped
A few strands of fresh **C**hives, finely cut with scissors
A large handful of **C**ashews, roasted

1. **Dressing:** In a screw-top glass jar, combine the ingredients. Screw the lid on and shake vigorously to mix well.
2. In a large bowl, combine the carrots and the herbs. Drizzle with some of the dressing. Toss, taste to adjust the seasoning, and top with cashews.

Thai Green Mango Salad

Serves 4-6
Prep Time: 15 min.
Cooking Time: optional grilling

Easy to prepare, and not only is it colourful, this salad is refreshing and fragrant.
The key to the distinctive appeal of this salad is the tartness of the under-ripe mangoes.

Salad:

2 large green or under ripe mangoes, peeled, seeded and julienned
1 carrot, peeled and julienned
1 red pepper, thinly sliced
½ green pepper, thinly sliced
¼ red onion, thinly sliced
¼ cup each coriander, mint and Thai basil leaves, cut in **chiffonade**☺
Optional: 1 cup of grilled shrimp or grilled chicken pieces

Dressing:

In a screw-top glass jar, combine the following ingredients. Screw the lid on and shake vigorously to blend. Taste and adjust the seasoning if needed.

Juice and zest of 1 lime
2 tbsp sucanat or coconut sugar (I often use maple syrup)
1 tbsp (or to taste) fish sauce
3 tbsp vegetable oil
½ tsp Sambal Oelek or other spicy chili sauce

To garnish: Fresh coriander, mint or Thai basil leaves
⅓ cup toasted cashews, chopped or whole

1. In a bowl, toss to combine mangoes, carrot, peppers, onion, ribbons of herbs and grilled shrimp or chicken.
2. Add the dressing and toss with the salad. Let stand for a few minutes to allow the flavours to marry.
3. Garnish with the herb leaves and the cashews.

☺How to make a **chiffonade:**

1. Wash fresh wide leaves like basil, mint or spinach, pat them dry with a paper towel.
2. Stack the leaves one on top of the other.
3. Roll the stack widthwise to create a long multi-layered tube.
4. With a sharp knife or scissors, slice or cut into long, thin ribbons across the tube. The thin ribbons are the chiffonade.

Visit my website at www.olivestolychees.com for a demonstration.

"You can't use up creativity.
The more you use, the more you have."
-Maya Angelou, U.S. author and poet

Salade niçoise

Serves 4-6
Prep Time: 40-45 min.
Cooking Time: 20 min.

This is a beautiful, composed salad that I like to serve year round because of the colourful goodness and… the tasty leftovers, cold or warmed up, the next day! Most *salades niçoises* that I have seen had all their ingredients tossed with the dressing. I prefer to arrange the ingredients on a large platter. I also like to add **grilled shrimp, grilled salmon, or pan-seared tuna** or a combination. You can also grill or bake a chicken breast or a piece of steak that you serve sliced and place in the middle of the vegetable display. The effect is quite appealing, and the guests can choose the ingredients they like. Feel free to present the salad in any way that would make your guests eat this complete dish.

Note: If don't like anchovies, you can omit them. I'll forgive you!

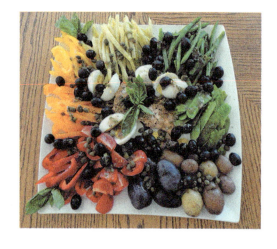

Salad:

½ lb each green and yellow string beans, ends trimmed, lightly cooked (or *al dente*)
½-¾ lb of baby new potatoes, white, red, purple, scrubbed, and cooked in salted water
4-5 hard-boiled eggs, peeled, quartered
The protein of your choice: fish, shrimp, meat
4-5 ripe tomatoes, quartered

1 red pepper, cut into strips
1 yellow pepper, cut into strips
1 orange pepper, cut into strips
1 green pepper, cut into strips
Any green vegetables, steamed until fork-tender, like asparagus, snow peas, sugar snaps

Garnishes:

½ red onion, thinly sliced
1 cup black olives, pitted
2 tbsp capers, rinsed and drained

3-4 tbsp fresh parsley, basil and chives, finely chopped
Celtic salt and pepper

Vinaigrette:

1 garlic clove, peeled
4 anchovy fillets, drained, finely chopped
Black pepper
½ tsp cane sugar

1 tsp fresh basil, finely chopped
2 tbsp white vinegar
4 tbsp olive oil

Salad:

Arrange the **Salad** ingredients attractively on a large platter. Sprinkle the first 3 **Garnishes** all over the **Salad** ingredients. Top with the herbs. Sprinkle salt and pepper.

Vinaigrette:

In a screw-top glass jar, combine all the ingredients. Screw the lid on and shake vigorously until creamy and emulsified. Taste and adjust the seasoning. Pour over the salad when ready to serve.

Variations:

- You can line the bottom and sides of the platter with romaine lettuce leaves to create a comfortable bed for the ingredients.
- This salad can also be made with leftover salmon, shrimp, roasted beef, and whatever raw, grilled or blanched vegetables. The quantity doesn't matter; use what you have on hand. The more varied the colours and the textures, the more impressive the salad will look and taste. Remember, we eat with our eyes first!

Greek Shrimp Salad

Serves 4
Prep Time: 20-30 min.
Cooking Time: 10 min.

An excellent menu item for a barbecue or picnic, this salad travels well. Just keep the dressing separately until you are ready to serve. The salad is even prettier with some slices of purple pepper, if you happen to find them.

Salad:

½ lb or 8-12 shrimp, shelled and deveined
Celtic salt and pepper
1 head romaine lettuce, washed and shredded, or various salad greens

4 small tomatoes, cut into wedges, or cherry tomatoes, whole or cut in half
1 medium English cucumber, halved lengthwise and sliced in half moons

½ red pepper, sliced
½ green pepper, sliced
½ orange pepper, sliced
½ yellow pepper, sliced
¼ red onion, finely sliced

1 cup of marinated artichokes, rinsed and drained (optional but very delicious)
1 cup of Kalamata olives (or any olives that you enjoy)
3½ oz Greek feta cheese, if desired
1 tbsp each fresh oregano and flat-leaf parsley, chopped

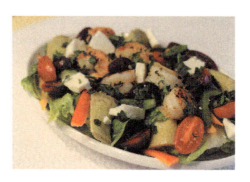

Dressing:

In a screw-top glass jar, combine the following ingredients. Screw the lid on and shake vigorously to emulsify.

3 tbsp olive oil
2 tbsp red wine vinegar
1 tbsp lemon juice
½ tsp lemon zest
1 tsp Dijon mustard

¼ tsp grated garlic
1 tsp cane sugar or maple syrup
Freshly chopped oregano
Salt and pepper

1. Season the shrimp with a little salt and pepper. In a pan, cook the shrimp until they turn pink on both sides. Reserve.
2. In a large salad bowl or in 4 bowls (or shallow containers, if you need to transport the salad), place the romaine pieces. On the lettuce pieces, arrange the vegetables, the olives, the feta, the herbs, and finally the shrimp. When ready to serve, drizzle the dressing over the salad.

*"A single act of kindness throws out roots in all directions,
and the roots spring up and make new trees."*
-Amelia Earhart, U.S. aviator

Sardinian Cauliflower

Serves 4
Prep Time: 20 min.
Cooking Time: 35 min.

It is a great way to use a whole cauliflower and turn it into a spectacular and colourful mound of goodness.

1 large whole cauliflower, green leaves removed
½ red pepper, finely chopped
¾ cup black or green pitted olives, sliced

¼ cup chopped parsley
Celtic salt and pepper
Olive oil

1. Place the whole cauliflower in a large pot of water. Add some salt and bring to a boil. Cover with a lid, reduce the heat and simmer gently for about 30-35 minutes, until tender.
2. Carefully lift the cauliflower out of the pot and place it onto a large platter, taking care not to break it. (If you do break it, don't worry about it; it will still be delicious and appealing.) Pile the red pepper and the olives on top. Sprinkle with parsley. Season with salt and pepper.
3. Drizzle with some olive oil. Serve warm by pulling out the florets.

Variations:

- If you don't want to cook the whole head, you can boil the florets individually, and toss them in a bowl with the rest of the ingredients.
- You can seed and finely chop 1 small tomato, and add it to the pile on top of the cauliflower.

Wilted Spinach with Fried Garlic

Serves 4
Prep Time: 10 min.
Cooking Time: 15 min.

For this side dish, it is best to use fresh spinach sold in bunches instead of the bagged variety. You can also use chard (red-leaf or regular) and remove the hard centre veins.

3 lbs fresh flat-leaf spinach, thoroughly washed
¼ cup olive oil
2 onions, thinly sliced
5-6 medium garlic cloves, cut in thin slices
Celtic salt and freshly ground black pepper
1 tbsp butter

1. Pat dry the washed spinach leaves. Cut the large leaves in half. Set aside.
2. Heat the oil in a large pan. Add the onion slices and sauté over medium heat until fragrant, about 5 minutes.
3. Stir in the garlic slices and cook until golden, about 2-3 minutes.
4. Add the spinach leaves to the pan. Stir them to coat with the oil. Season with salt and pepper to taste. Cover and cook, stirring a few times, until the leaves have wilted, 3-4 minutes. Remove the cover and simmer until some of the liquid has evaporated and the leaves are moist, 2-3 minutes. Serve immediately.

*"Never regret. If it's good, it's wonderful.
If it's bad, it's experience."*
-Victoria Holt, author

Greek Vegetable Kebabs

Serves 4
Prep Time: 15-20 min.
Cooking Time: 10 min.

Easy to prepare and quick to grill, these skewers are a must for any backyard barbecue menu! For the most flavours, allow the vegetables to marinate for more than 2 hours, preferably overnight. If you plan on using wooden skewers, they will have to be soaked in water for ½ hour prior to grilling to prevent scorching and burning. Using metal skewers is often more practical.

3 medium zucchinis, sliced lengthwise, then in 1-inch half-moons
1 large red pepper, seeded and cut into 1-inch squares
1 large yellow pepper, seeded and cut into 1-inch squares
1 large green pepper, seeded and cut into 1-inch" squares
1 medium red onion, peeled and cut in wedges
16-20 white mushrooms

Marinade:

Combine the following ingredients in a screw-top glass jar. Screw the lid and shake vigorously.

¾ cup olive oil
¼ cup white wine vinegar
1 garlic clove, minced
1 tsp each of Dijon mustard and coconut sugar
½ tsp each of basil, oregano, parsley, marjoram, and rosemary
¼ tsp ground black pepper

1. Place all the vegetables in a large Ziploc plastic bag. Add the marinade, seal the bag well. Move the bag from side to side to coat the vegetables. Refrigerate for at least 2 hours or overnight. Turn the bag over once in a while to redistribute the marinade over the vegetables.
2. When ready to grill, remove the vegetables from the bag, drain them, reserving the marinade. Using metal or pre-soaked wooden skewers, thread vegetables, alternating the colourful varieties.
3. Cook on a lightly greased grill over low heat, turning often and basting with the reserved marinade for about 10-15 minutes. Sprinkle with Celtic salt before serving.

Greek Roasted Potatoes

Serves 6
Prep Time: 10 min.
Cooking Time: 1 hour

If you are having kebabs or Souvlaki, you *need* to make these potatoes to go with them!
My condo neighbour Gary Bennett was happy to share this delicious recipe that he flavours with *Herbes de Provence*.
To accompany the kebabs, I created a Greek version with lemon and rosemary or oregano.

3 lbs red potatoes, scrubbed, quartered, and patted dry
A few glugs of olive oil
Celtic salt and pepper

1 tbsp of lemon zest
1 small sprig of fresh rosemary and/
or Greek oregano, finely chopped

Preheat oven to 400°F. Place potatoes in a baking sheet and toss them with olive oil, salt and pepper. Roast for 45 minutes. Toss and turn the potatoes once in a while, until they are golden brown, crisp on the outside and tender in the inside. Remove from the oven and sprinkle with the lemon zest and chopped herb. If you want a stronger lemon flavour, drizzle some lemon juice.

*"There are three things that cannot be hidden very long:
the sun, the moon, and… the truth."*
-Buddha

Greek Village Salad

Serves 6-8
Prep Time: 15 min.

This colourful salad is often called the "peasant salad" throughout Greece. If you are going to have kebabs or Souvlaki, you *need* a Greek salad to go with them! Serve it in a large salad bowl or in individual bowls. If you happen to find a rare purple pepper, adding it to this rainbow-like salad would look (and taste) amazing. Your guests will definitely notice the great eye appeal of this dish.

Salad:

½ small red onion, thinly sliced
1 English cucumber, chopped

2-3 tomatoes, quartered
1 red pepper, coarsely chopped

1 orange pepper, coarsely chopped
1 yellow pepper, coarsely chopped
1 green pepper, coarsely chopped
½ cup Kalamata olives

Optional: 5 oz Greek feta cheese, cubed or crumbled
To garnish: a small handful of fresh parsley, chopped; and a smaller handful of oregano, chopped

Dressing:

Combine the following ingredients in a screw-top glass jar.
Screw the lid on and shake vigorously. Taste and adjust the seasoning if necessary.

¼ cup olive oil
2 tbsp lemon juice
2 tbsp red or white wine vinegar
½ tsp Dijon mustard
1½ tsp dried Greek oregano (or 1 tbsp fresh Greek oregano)
Celtic salt and pepper to taste

1. Combine all the vegetables in a bowl. Scatter the olives and the feta, if using. Garnish with the herbs.
2. When ready to serve, pour the dressing over the salad and toss to coat.

Variations:

- For added crunch, you could add a few cups of torn romaine lettuce or baby arugula to the mix.
- You could add 1 tsp mashed anchovies (2-3 fillets) in the dressing.

Did you know that the traditional chef's hat originated in Greece?

Green Beans with Pancetta and Fried Shallots

Serves 4-6
Prep Time: 15-20 min.
Cooking Time: 15-20 min.

A tasty and simple combination of salty and spicy, this side dish can be made quickly for any weekday dinners.

1 lb green bean (also called *haricots verts*), trimmed
4-6 thin slices of pancetta, finely chopped
1 tbsp vegetable oil

Dressing:

In a screw-top glass jar, combine the following ingredients. Screw the lid on and shake vigorously.

1 tbsp red wine vinegar,
1 tbsp olive oil,
½ tsp fresh rosemary or thyme, finely chopped,
a good pinch of hot pepper flakes.

2 large shallots, peeled and cut into ⅛-inch thick rings (about 2 cups). Careful! They might make you cry!
4-5 tbsp vegetable oil or more

1. In a large pot, bring some salted water to a boil. Boil the beans until *al dente* (or still crunchy), about 4 minutes.
2. While the beans are cooking, you can assemble the dressing.
3. Drain and cool the beans under cold water. Drain again and set aside. If you prefer to steam the beans, go right ahead. This step can be done up to 2 days ahead. The cooked beans can be refrigerated in an airtight container. They will need to be warmed up before assembly time.
4. In a skillet, heat up the oil over medium heat; add the pancetta pieces and cook until crisp, 5-7 minutes. Transfer to cool on a paper towel-lined platter.
5. In the skillet, heat up the 4-5 tbsp of oil over medium heat until hot. In small handfuls, gently ease the shallot rings into the oil, stirring occasionally with a wooden spoon until they are golden, about 1-2 minutes. Transfer to a paper towel-lined platter and season with Celtic salt and pepper.
6. **Assembly:** In a mixing bowl, toss the warmed beans, the cooked pancetta and the dressing together. Transfer to a serving platter, and top with the fried shallot rings. Season with salt and pepper to taste.

"If there's nobody in your way,
it's because you're not going anywhere."
-Unknown

Roasted Sicilian Cauliflower

Serves 4
Prep Time: 15 min.
Cooking Time: 40 min.

Roasting anything transforms its flavours as it enhances the umami taste to a level that is rich and savory.

1 whole cauliflower, cut into florets	¼ cup raisins
olive oil	¼ cup toasted pine nuts
2-3 thin slices of prosciutto	2 tbsp ground flaxseeds
1 garlic clove, minced or grated with a microplane	Zest and juice of ½ lemon
1-2 tbsp capers, rinsed and drained	Ground black pepper to taste

1. Preheat oven to 425°F. In a bowl, toss the florets with 2 tbsp oil. Spread on a baking sheet. Line another baking sheet with parchment paper, and arrange the prosciutto slices on top.
2. Put both baking sheets in the oven, the cauliflower to roast and the prosciutto to crisp. Keep an eye on both, especially the prosciutto so it doesn't burn or trigger your smoke detector. Flip the prosciutto slices over after a few minutes. Remove when they are crisp and dry. Let cool; then, break into bite-size pieces.
3. Occasionally, stir the cauliflower until it is crispy and golden, in about 30-40 minutes.
4. When the cauliflower is roasted, transfer to a serving bowl. Mix in the garlic, capers, raisins, prosciutto pieces, and pine nuts. Spoon some flaxseeds over the top. Sprinkle the lemon zest and squeeze some lemon juice over the top. Season with some black pepper (no salt, as the prosciutto is already salty) and serve warm.

Other Roasting Ideas

The method is the same for all vegetables: Preheat the oven between 400-450°F. Prepare the vegetables and cut into chunks. Toss in a baking pan with olive oil, Celtic salt and pepper. You can also include some finely chopped fresh herbs. Roast, turning occasionally until the vegetables are tender and caramelized. Since you have the oven on, you might as well roast a few different vegetables. You will be happy you did. Enjoy, this is great food that will make your kitchen smell lovely where everyone will want to be! RT = Roasting Time

Choices of vegetables:

Beets Oven: 450°F, RT: 1 h. Roast wrapped in a foil packet. Cool and remove the skins. Delicious in salad with some creamy cheese, like blue cheese.
Bell Peppers Oven: 500°F, RT: ¼ h. Roast cut side down until charred. Let cool in a paper bag or covered in plastic wrap. Slip off and discard the skins. Delicious in salad, sandwiches, soups, etc.
Carrots Oven: 400°F, RT: ½ h. Great accompaniment to a meat dish.
Garlic Oven: 425°F, RT: 30-40 min. Roast covered in foil. Let cool. Squeeze the cloves out of their skins. When roasted, garlic has a sweet and nutty flavour. Delightful as a spread on bread or crackers.
Puréed Onion Oven: 400°F, RT: ¾ h. Before roasting, cut into wedges, leaving root ends intact; peel. Cool and purée until smooth. Great as a spread. Don't want a purée? Serve the wedges with other roasted vegetables, grilled or roasted meats.
Potatoes Oven: 425°F, RT: ½ h. Scrub and dry before roasting. They can be served hot or cold. Wonderful in salads, or as an accompaniment to a meat dish.
Zucchini Oven: 450°F, RT: ¼ h. Cut into 1-inch thick rounds. Lovely as a side dish, or in a roasted vegetable salad.

Thai Beef Salad

Serves 4
Prep Time: 20-30 min.
Cooking Time: 5 min.

Cooked chicken or shrimp can be substituted for the beef. You can even combine them.
The colourful ingredients make this salad very appealing.

Salad:

1 head of romaine lettuce, shredded
1 lb sirloin steak
Sesame oil
1 kaffir lime leaf, centre vein removed, finely chopped
¼ cup each of basil and mint, finely chopped
⅓ cup coriander, finely chopped
¼ small red onion, thinly sliced

½ English cucumber, peeled and julienned
1 large handful of snow peas, trimmed and julienned
¼ small red pepper, finely diced
¼ small Chinese cabbage, shredded
1 small handful of bean sprouts
A handful of chives, chopped
¼ cup roasted cashews, chopped

Dressing:

In a screw-top glass jar, combine the following ingredients. Screw the lid on and shake vigorously. Taste and adjust the seasoning, if needed.
¼ cup vegetable oil
2-3 tbsp sesame oil

2 tbsp fish sauce
½ tsp hot pepper flakes or Sambal Oelek
Juice of 1 lime
2 tsp maple syrup

1. Line a large platter with the romaine lettuce.
2. Brush the steak with the oil and pan-fry over high heat until cooked to your liking. Transfer to a plate and let it rest, covered with foil, for a few minutes before slicing very thinly.
3. In a large mixing bowl, combine the rest of the salad ingredients. Add the steak slices and mix well. Pour the dressing over the salad, toss to coat. Serve at room temperature.

Steamed Vegetables with Tomato Dressing

Serves 4
Prep Time: 10 min.
Cooking time: 10 min.

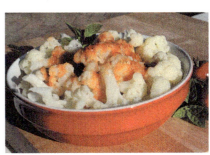

Inspired by the brilliant Jamie Oliver, I often make this simple and healthy dressing to be drizzled over steaming hot vegetables. To make the dressing, you will need a microplane or a fine grater.

Dressing:

1 tomato, cut in half
¼ of a small red onion
1 garlic clove

Zest and juice of ½ lemon or ½ orange
Olive oil
Celtic salt and pepper

½ cauliflower head and/or broccoli head, cut in florets

1. Over a small bowl to collect all the juices, grate the tomato halves, the onion, the garlic, and the lemon zest. Add the lemon juice and a few glugs (about 3 tbsp or so) of olive oil. Season with salt and pepper. Whisk to combine. Taste and adjust the seasoning if needed. Set aside.

2. Steam the cauliflower and/or broccoli florets until tender but still *al dente*. Transfer to a serving bowl. Drizzle the dressing over the hot vegetables and toss to coat. Serve while warm.

Variation:

For a Thai flavour, I use lime instead of lemon, grate some gingerroot, and garnish with chopped basil.

Spinach Salad with Red Grapes and Smoked Salmon Roses

Serves 4-6
Prep Time: 10-15 min.

A pretty and colourful salad with a salty-smoky-sweet flavour; this is sure to impress!

Salad:

6 cups baby spinach leaves, washed, dried
2 cups red seedless grapes, cut in half
1 green onion, sliced
1 orange pepper, seeded and diced
½ lb smoked salmon, cut in slices
1-2 tbsp capers, rinsed and drained

Vinaigrette:

In a screw-top glass jar, combine the vinaigrette ingredients. Screw the lid on and shake vigorously until well combined and emulsified. Keep the unused portion refrigerated.
1 tsp Dijon mustard
1 tbsp sucanat or maple syrup
2 tbsp white wine vinegar
4 tbsp olive oil
2-3 tbsp fresh dill, chopped
Freshly grounded black pepper

Salad: Place the spinach leaves in a large salad bowl. Add the grapes, green onion and orange pepper. Pour a small amount of vinaigrette over and gently toss to coat. Distribute the salad in 4 to 6 serving plates. Garnish each plate with a few smoked salmon roses.

Salmon roses: Roll a slice of salmon lengthwise, gather the layers of one side while spreading open the layers of the opposite side, creating the leaves of a rose. Repeat with the remaining salmon slices. Insert some capers inside the roses. Drizzle each salad with a thin stream of vinaigrette. Serve immediately.

Salade de légumes marinés
(Marinated Vegetable Salad)

Serves 4-6
Prep Time: 20 min.
Cooking Time: 10 min.
Chilling Time: 1-2 hours

I like to bring this salad to pot-luck parties and picnics because it can be prepared ahead of time. No reheating is required and it travels well.

½ cauliflower, cut into florets
½ broccoli, cut into florets
1 carrot, peeled and cut in thin slices
½ lb each of green beans and yellow wax beans, trimmed, cut in half
½ sweet red pepper, seeded and cut into chunks
¼ small red onion, thinly sliced
½ cup of pitted olives (green, black or Kalamata)
1 cup cherry tomatoes

Dressing:

In a screw-top glass jar, combine all ingredients. Screw the lid on and shake vigorously.

3 tbsp olive oil	½ tsp dried oregano
3 tbsp cider vinegar	½ tsp dried rosemary
1 tsp Dijon mustard	1 tsp Celtic salt
1 tsp maple syrup	½ tsp ground black pepper
1 garlic clove, minced	**To garnish:** fresh parsley and basil, chopped

1. In a pot, boil some water with 1 tsp salt. Add cauliflower and the broccoli florets; cover and cook until crisp, 2-3 minutes. Transfer to a large bowl.
2. Add carrots and beans to the boiling water; cover and cook until crisp, 2-3 minutes or less. Transfer to the large bowl.
3. In the large bowl, add the peppers, olives, and red onion. Stir to combine. Pour the dressing over the vegetables and stir to mix. Refrigerate for 1-2 hours, stirring occasionally.
4. To serve, toss in the cherry tomatoes, and garnish with the chopped herbs.

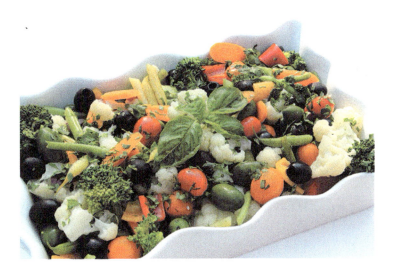

Flying Protein

Chicken and Turkey

Bok-Bok-Bok!

Who doesn't like chicken?
It is such a popular protein choice everywhere in the world, and on all restaurant menus.
It is easy to raise, to cook, and it provides tasty lean meat.

I am so grateful that more and more regular grocery stores are now selling properly fed, hormone- and antibiotic-free organic chicken, at a reasonable price, and in a wider selection of cuts: "whole bird", breasts, thighs, drumsticks, even wings!

I often buy the whole bird that I roast, or cook *"en crapaudine"* ("like a frog"; I cut it alongside its backbone, turn it over, flatten it on the breast bone and lay it cut side down in a baking dish.) Or I poach it in a large stockpot in plenty of water, vegetables, herbs and spices that give juicy meat and a delicious stock for multiple uses later.

With a whole bird, there are many cooking options and derived meals.
It is like cooking once and having several meals almost ready to go.

As I do not find organic turkey very often, I use mostly chicken. For the following recipes, you could easily substitute turkey parts, if you would prefer, or even duck, goose, ostrich or whatever other flying (or winged) protein you like or feel tempted to experiment with.

Go for it and ... **soar!**

*"Nothing would be more tiresome than eating and drinking
if God had not made them a pleasure as well as a necessity."*
-Voltaire, French philosopher

No-fuss Baked Chicken Dinner

Serves 4
Prep Time: 10-15 min.
Cooking Time: 35-40 min.

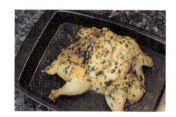

This no-fuss dinner is my saviour when I don't have time or the inspiration to make anything more elaborate, and Philip wants chicken! It is tasty, juicy and healthy. If I want to, I save the leftover meat and flavourful broth to make a Chicken Soup the next day, which he loves. It is a quick and satisfying meal to prepare because, while the chicken is cooking, I can steam 2 to 3 vegetables and make a green salad. So, dinner can be served in less than 45 minutes!

4-6 chicken legs or thighs or a combination, bone-in, excess fat removed, washed
Juice of ½ lemon (orange juice works, too)
Celtic salt and pepper
Pinches of dried herbs of your choice like parsley, basil, oregano

1 tsp dehydrated onion flakes
1 garlic clove, chopped
Pinch of hot red pepper
Zest of ½ lemon (orange zest is great, too)
3 cups chicken broth

Optional Extras: ¼ cup sun-dried tomatoes, chopped; 1 small carrot, diced; 1 celery stalk, diced

1. Preheat the oven to 350°F.
2. In a shallow baking dish, place the chicken pieces, cut side down for the thighs.
3. Drizzle the lemon juice over the chicken pieces. Season with salt and pepper. Scatter all the herbs, onion flakes, garlic, red pepper, and zest.
4. Pour the broth around the chicken pieces to create a nice bath.
5. If you like, you can add the **optional extras** for additional flavour.
6. Cover with aluminum foil and bake for 35-40 minutes, or until the juices run clear (instead of pink) when you pierce a thigh or a leg near the bone with a knife.
7. Remove from the oven, let rest, covered, for a few minutes.

Variation:

I like to use a **whole chicken** that I cook *en crapaudine*. For a demonstration, visit my website at www.olivestolychees.com.

Here is what you can do:

Place the chicken breast side down on a cutting board. With a pair of kitchen scissors or a sharp chef's knife, remove the backbone by cutting on either side of it or cut on only one side and leave the rest of the backbone attached. This will allow you to open the chicken like a book. Then, turn the chicken over on the cut side. Place your hands on the breast bone and flatten the chest. Place the flattened chicken in a baking dish. To flavour the skin, rub a grated **garlic clove** and the **zest of a lemon** over it, season with **salt and pepper**. Drizzle some **olive oil** and **lemon juice**, and sprinkle **chopped herbs** like basil or rosemary. Finally, pour a little bit of **chicken broth** or water to cover the bottom of the dish. Bake at 375°F, for 30-40 minutes, occasionally basting with the pan juices, adding more broth if needed. Bake until fragrant and, when you pierce the thigh with a knife, the juices run clear instead of pink. Let it rest, covered, for 15 minutes before serving.

Chicken Tagine with Olives and Preserved Lemons
(Adapted from Ghillie Başan's recipes in her book *Flavors of Morocco*.)

Serves 4-6
Prep Time: 15 min.
Chilling Time: 1- 2 hours
Cooking Time: about 1 hour

Another Moroccan classic dish that is flavoured with two of the most traditional ingredients: preserved lemons and cracked green olives. Both ingredients can be purchased at Middle Eastern stores and gourmet shops. The tagine can be made with chicken thighs and/or drumsticks or a whole chicken. Traditionally served over couscous, this dish would feel equally satisfying if served with a steamed vegetable dish or a colourful side salad like the ones from the previous chapter.

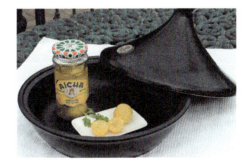

Pictured on the right is the flameproof earthenware *tagine* with its pointed lid used to cook many Moroccan stews.

This is the jar of preserved lemons that I particularly like because it only contains lemon, water and salt.

Marinade:

Combine all the ingredients in a bowl.
1 onion, peeled and grated
2 garlic cloves, peeled, grated
A 1-inch piece of ginger, peeled and grated
A large handful of fresh coriander, finely chopped
A pinch of saffron

½ tsp hot pepper flakes
Juice of 1 lemon
1 tsp Celtic salt
3-4 tbsp olive oil
1 tsp black pepper

Chicken

8-12 chicken thighs and/or drumsticks	1½ cups cracked green olives
1 tbsp oil + 1 tbsp butter	1 tsp each of dried oregano and dried thyme
Water or chicken broth	Harissa or hot pepper sauce to serve
2 preserved lemons, cut into strips	

1. Place the chicken pieces in a shallow glass dish; coat with the marinade, rubbing it into the skin. Cover and chill for 1-2 hours.
2. In a tagine or a Dutch oven, heat the oil and butter over medium heat. Remove the chicken pieces from the marinade and brown them in oil for a few minutes.
3. Pour over the marinade left in the dish; add enough water or broth to come halfway up the sides of the chicken pieces. Bring the liquid to a boil; reduce the heat, cover with a lid, and gently simmer for about 45 minutes, occasionally turning the pieces over.
4. Add the preserved lemons, olives, and half the herbs to the tagine. Cover, and simmer for 15-20 minutes more. Check the seasoning. Sprinkle with the rest of the herbs over the top. Serve with some harissa or hot sauce on the side.

Moroccan Chicken Stew

Serves 4
Prep Time: 20 min.
Cooking Time: about 1 hour

This stew is great served over sweet potato mash.
The exotic spice mix is warming and makes this dish a perfect one for a winter dinner.

¼ tsp each of ground cinnamon, cloves and hot pepper flakes	2 cups chicken broth
½ tsp each of ground coriander, cumin and turmeric	1 tbsp each of lemon zest and juice
8-10 chicken thighs, bone-in, trimmed of excess fat	1 preserved lemon rind, finely chopped
2 tbsp olive oil	(preserved lemon can be purchased in jars at Middle-Eastern food stores)
2 onion, finely chopped	¼ cup green olives, pitted and cut in half
2 garlic cloves, finely chopped	2 tbsp each of fresh parsley and coriander, chopped

1. In a large bowl, combine the spices. Add the thighs and coat well with the spices.
2. In an oven-proof skillet or pan, heat the oil over medium heat. Working in small batches, add a few of the chicken thighs and brown on all sides. When cooked, transfer to a plate and continue cooking the rest of the thighs.
3. Add more oil if necessary to cook the onions until softened, stirring to dislodge the caramelized chicken bits adhering to the bottom of the pan. Add the garlic and cook for a minute or so.
4. Return the chicken to the pan. Add the broth, lemon zest and juice. Bring to a boil; then, reduce the heat to a simmer. Cook, covered until fragrant for about 35-45 minutes.
5. Transfer the thighs to a serving bowl and cover with a piece of foil to keep warm. You may keep them warm in the oven set at its lowest temperature.
6. Bring the liquid to a boil to create a richer sauce. Add the lemon rind and the olives. Simmer for 8-10 minutes until slightly thickened.
7. Pour over the chicken thighs and garnish with the chopped herbs.

Coq au vin
(French Chicken Stew in Red Wine)

Serves 4-6
Prep Time: 20 min.
Cooking Time: about 1½ hours

"Coq" is French for *cock* or *rooster*. It is now used as a synonym for chicken in certain dishes. In traditional stock farming, cocks that were good breeders were kept as long as they could fulfil their function. They would be several years old before they were killed and, therefore, needed long and slow braising in wine. Nowadays, *"coq au vin"* is usually made with a chicken or a hen. A perfect cold winter night dinner served with mashed roots, this meal is praise worthy.

½ lb bacon or pancetta, cut in small pieces
3-4 lbs of chicken thighs and/or drumsticks, washed and patted dry
1 large onion, peeled and diced
2 carrots, peeled and diced
1 celery, diced
2 garlic cloves, minced
2-3 cup chicken broth
¼ cup Cognac or Brandy

1 bottle of red wine like Burgundy
1 fresh sprig of thyme
3 carrots, peeled, cut into chunks
2 dozen pearl onions☺
2 tbsp butter
1 lb cremini or white mushrooms, stems removed and quartered
Celtic salt and pepper
Chopped parsley to garnish

1. Preheat the oven to 275°F. In a large Dutch oven, heat some oil over medium heat. Add the bacon or pancetta. Cook until lightly browned, about 10 minutes. With a slotted spoon, transfer to a paper towel-lined plate.
2. Season the chicken pieces with salt and pepper. In small batches, add the chicken pieces in the hot Dutch oven and brown for a few minutes, turning on all sides for even browning. When browned, transfer to a plate. Continue cooking the rest of the chicken. Set aside on the plate.
3. Add the diced onion, carrots, celery; season with salt and pepper; cook, stirring occasionally, over medium heat for 10 minutes or so until the onion have softened and are golden. Add the garlic and cook for about 1 minute. Add 1 cup of chicken broth. Bring to a boil and scrape any food bits that have adhered to the bottom of the pot. Simmer for a few minutes to further cook the carrots and celery. With a hand-held blender, purée the mixture to a smooth consistency. Since we are not using any flour as a thickening agent, puréeing the mixture will create the rich sauce needed for this stew.
4. Raise the heat again. Add the Cognac or Brandy and let the alcohol burn off. Return the bacon or pancetta, chicken and any juices accumulated in the plate to the pot. Add the wine, remaining chicken stock, thyme, carrots, and pearl onions; bring to a boil.
5. Cover the pot with a lid and transfer to the oven. Cook for 30-45 minutes, until the chicken pieces, when pierced with a knife near a bone, are no longer pink, and the carrots are tender.
6. While the *coq au vin* is cooking, in a sauté pan, melt the butter over medium heat. Cook the mushrooms until browned, about 20-25 minutes. Add to the stew in the last 10 minutes of cooking. Remove from the oven. Check the seasoning and adjust it if necessary.
7. Serve in bowls garnished with fresh chopped parsley.

☺ To easily peel the pearl onions (without any tears!), put them in a bowl and pour some very hot water over them. Let them soak for 20 minutes. Using a knife, you can cut the stems off, and the skins will come off quite easily.

Chinese Chicken Hot Pot
(or Asian Fondue)

Serves 4
Prep Time: 20-30 min.
Cooking Time: 2-4 min. at the table

I love to prepare fun and interactive hot pots or fondue for friends; the type of meal that allows us to talk for hours and eat leisurely. I also like this relaxed and intimate setting to celebrate a special occasion with just Philip and me. This meal is special enough for a celebration, yet healthy and "**clean**" enough to be considered **spa food**.

Use an assortment of meat, fish and seafood that provide a good variety of colours and textures. The broth, the dippers, and the dipping sauce can be prepared ahead of time and kept chilled in separate containers until required. Even though this recipe is in the **Flying Protein (chicken)** chapter, I have included meat, fish and seafood in the ingredient list. I had to insert the recipe somewhere!

Broth:

- 4 cups of chicken stock
- 1 small hot red pepper, seeded and crushed
- 1 tbsp ginger, peeled and grated
- 2 garlic cloves, peeled and crushed
- 2 shallots, peeled and chopped
- 3 star anise
- 2 tsp honey
- 1 tsp black peppercorns
- 1 tbsp fresh coriander, finely chopped

Protein Dippers:

- ½ lb chicken breast, cut in strips
- ½ lb sirloin steak, cut in strips
- ½ lb fresh shrimp, shelled and deveined
- ½ lb fresh scallops, each sliced in half to create 2 thin disks
- ½ lb fresh salmon, cut into cubes or strips

Vegetable Dippers:

- 1 medium zucchini, cut into strips
- 1 red bell pepper, seeded and cut into strips
- 1 yellow red pepper, seeded and cut into strips
- 8 white mushrooms, stems removed
- A head of broccoli, cut in florets
- A dozen baby bok choi
- A dozen cherry tomatoes
- 1 cup bean sprouts
- Fresh coriander leaves to garnish

Dipping sauce:

- 1 tsp sesame oil
- 3 tbsp organic tamari
- 1 tsp honey
- ½ tsp hot red pepper or Sambal Oelek
- 2 tsp dry sherry

Garnishing:

- Chopped coriander
- Hot red pepper

1. **Broth:** Prepare the broth on the stove by combining all broth ingredients in a saucepan; bring to a boil; then, simmer for about 10 minutes. Transfer to a fondue pot, and place over the lit burner.
2. **Dippers:** On a platter, arrange the **protein dippers**. On a separate platter, arrange the **vegetable dippers**. Garnish each platter with fresh coriander leaves.
3. **Dipping Sauce:** In a screw-top glass jar, combine the dipping sauce ingredients. Screw the lid on, shake vigorously and transfer to 4 small bowls.
4. Provide each diner with a fondue fork. Each diner spears a protein and a vegetable dipper, and dips it in the hot broth for 2-4 minutes. When all the dippers have been cooked, add the bean sprouts to the broth. Heat for a few minutes; then, serve the broth as a soup, garnished with coriander and hot red pepper, if desired.
5. Take your time and have fun. This is great food. Everyone will enjoy their own cooking!

Grazing Protein

Beef and Lamb

At different times in my life, I chose a vegetarian and a vegan lifestyle for various reasons: as a university student and a freshly hired teacher, I could not afford buying meat; a few years ago, I couldn't stomach it.

I am not a vegetarian at the moment; however, I choose to consume less meat and fish.
I prefer to explore new and delicious ways to prepare the freshest and ripest produce I find at the market.

About a year ago, I met a farmer whose practices, ethics and products I can trust. I have been buying his organic meats and I thoroughly enjoy them. I find the texture, the smell when it is being cooked and the flavours once cooked much more appealing than the conventional option. It smells and tastes like real meat! Many people avoid eating red meat.
I feel that we only need to keep in mind 3 key words:
gratitude -- for the animal's sacrifice and the farmer's care,
quality -- from a good organic source, whenever possible,
and **quantity** -- using the meat pieces as a flavouring for a dish.

Personally, I only need a few bites to feel satisfied. I often choose fresh New Zealand spring lamb meat because the animals are allowed to roam around outside and eat grass. If you don't like lamb, you can substitute beef or pork or other red meats.

After a long flight at high altitude (too much Air element from a Polarity Therapy point of view), I particularly appreciate a small piece of beef (a food from the Earth element in Polarity Therapy) to ground myself faster, cope with the jetlag effects, and get acclimatized with the surroundings and the local time.

(For more information on the elements and Polarity Therapy, please refer to **Volume 2** of *Olives to Lychees, Everyday Mediter-asian Spa Cuisine* or visit my website at www.mindyourbodyandspirit.com.)

Do you know why a cooked roast needs to rest for about 15 minutes before carving?
To allow the natural juices to be re-absorbed.

Moroccan Tagine of Lamb, Vegetables and Prunes

Serves 6
Prep Time: 45-50 min.
Cooking Time: 1¾ hours

The aromatic and sweet flavours of this slow-cooked, hearty dish are quite comforting on a cold day. They form the basis of traditional Moroccan cooking. This dish is usually cooked in a vessel called *tagine* – a flameproof dish made of glazed earthenware with its matching cone cover. The *tagine* is used to cook Moroccan stews of meat, fish, poultry or vegetables. The vessel and the stews are both called *tagines*. The servings are traditionally served over steamed couscous made of durum semolina; however, you could ladle the portions over mashed sweet potatoes instead. If you don't have a tagine to cook the stew in, you can use a heavy-based pot or Dutch oven.

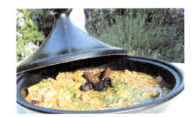

¼ cup olive oil
2 lbs lamb or beef, cut in small cubes
Celtic salt and pepper
½ tsp each of ground cinnamon and ginger

2 tsp ground cumin
1 tsp ground turmeric
1 large onion, finely chopped
2 cloves garlic, crushed

2-3 carrots, peeled, cut into ½-inch pieces	¾ cup pitted prunes, halved
1 zucchini, cut into 1-inch pieces	1 tbsp honey (optional)
2¾ cups water	2 tbsp fresh coriander, chopped
A pinch of saffron threads	½ cup blanched almonds, toasted
2 strips of orange rind	2 tbsp sesame seeds, toasted
1-2 cinnamon sticks	A handful of fresh coriander leaves, chopped

1. In a Dutch oven, heat oil over medium-high heat. Season the lamb cubes with salt and pepper. Add to the pot with the ground spices; cook, stirring, until the cubes are browned all over. Remove from the pot; set aside in a bowl.
2. Add onion and garlic to the pot and cook, stirring for a few minutes. Add carrots and cook for a few minutes. Add the zucchini and cook for a minute. Season with salt and pepper.
3. Stir in the water, saffron, orange rind and cinnamon stick(s). Return lamb cubes to the pot. Bring to a boil as you scrape the sides and bottom of the pot to dislodge the caramelized bits of goodness; then, simmer, covered, for 1 hour or until the lamb is tender.
4. Stir in the prunes, honey (if using), and coriander. Simmer, covered, for about 30 minutes, or until the carrots are tender. Remove the cinnamon stick and orange rind. Serve the tagine sprinkled with almonds, sesame seeds and fresh coriander leaves.

Variation:

You could create various versions of this tagine with different vegetables (butternut squash, parsnip, peppers, etc.) and dried fruit (apricots, dates and figs).

Greek Souvlaki and Tzatziki

Serves 6
Prep Time: 15-20 min.
Chilling Time: 3 hours
Cooking Time: 5-10 min.

The intoxicating aroma of meat kebabs being grilled on the barbecue is absolutely irresistible! The flavour of these kebabs will be further enhanced when you marinate them for at least a few hours, even overnight. Serve them with **Roasted Potatoes**, the **Vegetable Kebabs** and the **Village Salad**, and you will have a complete Greek meal. You can find these recipes in the **Loading Up on the Greens (Salads and Vegetables Dishes)** section. If you are using wooden skewers, they will need to soak in water for ½ hour prior to grilling to prevent scorching and burning.

Marinade

½ cup olive oil	2 garlic cloves, minced
1 cup red wine	2 tsp dry oregano
Juice of 1 lemon	Celtic salt and pepper

3 lbs of meat, cut into 1½-inch cubes (lamb, beef, pork, chicken, or a combination)

To garnish: dry oregano and lemon wedges

1. Mix the marinade ingredients in a glass bowl. Add the meat cubes, toss to coat well.
2. Cover and refrigerate for 3 hours or more. Stir the cubes once in a while to ensure even coating.
3. Half an hour before grilling, take the meat cubes out of the refrigerator to warm up a little.
4. Thread the meat cubes on the skewers; reserve the marinade.
5. Grill the skewers on the barbecue or under the broiler about 6" from the heat source. Turn the skewers once or twice while brushing with the marinade. Grill or broil until the desired degree of doneness is achieved, between 5 and 10 minutes, depending on your barbecue or broiler. Sprinkle with oregano. Serve with lemon wedges and **Tzatziki**.

Tzatziki☺

Makes 1 cup
1 medium English cucumber, peeled, seeded and shredded
½ tsp Celtic salt
½ cup plain Greek yogurt
½ tsp garlic clove minced

1 tsp fresh dill, finely chopped
1 tsp fresh mint, finely chopped
1 tsp extra-virgin olive oil
1 tsp lemon juice
½ tsp salt

1. In a colander, toss together cucumber and salt. Place the colander in the sink and let drain for ½ hour.
2. Press on the cucumber to extract excess liquid. Transfer to a bowl and mix in yogurt, garlic, dill, mint, oil, lemon juice, and salt.
3. Refrigerate about 1 hour to marry the flavours. Serve at room temperature.

☺If you want to make this dip dairy free, use 1 ripe avocado, increase the lemon juice and olive oil, and blend in a blender or with a hand-held blender. Taste and adjust the flavour to your palate.

Osso Buco alla Milanese
(Braised Veal Shanks)

Serves 4
Prep Time: 30-40 min.
Cooking Time: About 4 hours

This is one of my favourite classic Italian meat dishes, comforting and delicious. Perfect for a weekend dinner with a salad, and steamed or roasted vegetables. I have also used lamb shanks and the end result was equally tasty: fork-tender meat, and a delicious sauce. It can be served with Potato Mash and a salad. See below for the **Optional Potato Mash** recipe. The cooking time seems long, but once the shanks are slowly cooking in the low-heat oven, you are free to do other things. It is truly worth the effort! I am sure that it will become one of your family's favourites!

Osso buco:

1-2 bay leaves
4 cloves
1 sprig of fresh rosemary
1 orange
1 lemon
4 veal or lamb shanks
1 tbsp Celtic salt
Olive oil

2 cups onion, finely chopped
½ cup carrot, peeled and shredded
½ cup celery, finely chopped
2 tsp tomato paste
1 cup canned San Marzano tomatoes, crushed
1½ cups white wine
6-7 cups chicken broth, heated
Salt and pepper to taste

Gremolata:

Combine these ingredients together:

2 tbsp fresh flat parsley or basil, finely chopped
1 garlic clove, finely chopped
Zests of half a lemon and half an orange

Optional Potato Mash:

5-7 large Yukon Gold potatoes, peeled and cubed
(can also include 1 sweet potato, peeled and cubed)
Celtic salt
3-4 tbsp butter

¼-⅓ cup milk
1 cup grated mozzarella
⅓ cup flaxseeds
Fresh parsley, chopped

1. Make a *bouquet garni* (or herb bundle): cut a small square of cheesecloth and wrap the bay leaves, cloves and rosemary. Tie with a piece of kitchen twine and set aside.
2. With a sharp knife or a vegetable peeler, remove wide strips of the lemon and the orange zests, taking care not to include the white and bitter pith. Set aside. Squeeze and strain the juice of the orange. Set aside.
3. To keep the shanks intact while cooking, it is a good idea to secure the meat around the bone by "tying a belt" tightly around the outside of each osso buco with a piece of kitchen twine. Season the meat with salt and pepper.
4. In a large Dutch oven, heat oil over medium-high heat. Place the shanks in the pot, and allow to cook for 4-5 minutes, until the bottoms are browned. With a pair of tongs, turn the shanks to brown on all sides. Take your time to allow the browning to create great flavours. When all shanks have been browned on all sides, transfer them to a platter.
5. Pour more oil in the Dutch oven and add the onions. Cook over medium-high heat. With your spoon, scrape around to release the bits of caramelized meat on the bottom of the pot. Stir in the carrot and celery. Add the *bouquet garni*, and sprinkle 1 tsp of salt. Cook, stirring, until the vegetables are sizzling and softening.
6. Preheat the oven to 325°F.
7. Move the vegetables away from the centre of the pot and drop in the tomato paste. Cook the paste for a minute; then, mix it with the vegetables. Stir in the crushed tomatoes, and bring to a boil. Raise the heat, pour the wine and cook for a few minutes at a boil to evaporate the alcohol. Pour in 5-6 cups of chicken broth and the orange juice. Add all the strips of lemon and orange zest, 1 tsp of salt, and bring to a boil.
8. Return the shanks to the Dutch oven and immerse them completely in the sauce, adding more broth to cover the tops of the shanks, if necessary. Cover the Dutch oven and transfer it to the preheated oven. Cook for an hour or so.
9. After an hour, check to see if the shanks are still covered with the liquid. Add more broth if needed. Flip the shanks over so the meat can cook evenly on both sides.
10. Cook for 2-3 hours, until the meat is fork tender, and the sauce has reduced and thickened. Turn off the oven.
11. While the shanks are being cooked, prepare the **Potato Mash**. In a large pot, boil the potatoes in salted water. Once cooked, drain them, and mash them with butter. Add milk and whip the mixture into a creamy, smooth consistency. Taste and season, if needed. Cover the bottom of a baking dish with half of the potato mash, smoothing the surface. Sprinkle some mozzarella, flaxseeds, and add the rest of the potato mash. Sprinkle more mozzarella and flaxseeds on top, and bake until golden and bubbling. Remove from oven and set aside. Cut into squares.
12. When the shanks are fork-tender, transfer them to a serving platter. Cut the twine and discard it. Lift the *bouquet garni*, press it against the side of the pot to release all the juices into the pot, and discard it.
13. With a hand-held immersion blender, purée the sauce to a thick and velvety texture. Taste the sauce and adjust the seasoning if needed.
14. To serve, place a shank in a soup bowl, spoon some sauce over it and sprinkle 1 tsp of **Gremolata** on top. Serve with a square of **Potato Mash**.

> *"Do what you can,*
> *with what you have,*
> *where you are."*
> -Theodore Roosevelt

Grilled Moroccan Lamb Skewers

Serves: 6
Prep: 20-25 min.
Cooking Time: 10 min.

Lamb is a very much appreciated meat in countries like Morocco, Algeria, Tunisia, and Greece. Cooking a whole lamb *rôtisserie*-style, or pit-roasted, outdoors, called *méchoui,* is a culinary event not to miss. The lamb is resting on a long stick, is brushed all over with melted butter flavoured with coarse salt and spices, and set over ashes to begin its long slow cooking. Once cooked, it is eaten with a spicy sauce called *harissa*. This sauce can be found in convenient tubes in most grocery stores, or it can be homemade. For this recipe, you will need skewers; if yours are wooden, they will have to be soaked in cold water for 30 minutes before grilling, to prevent scorching and burning.

1 tbsp cumin seeds
2 lb ground lamb (use ground beef if you can't find ground lamb, or if you don't like lamb)
1 onion, finely chopped
2 garlic cloves, minced
½ tsp fresh parsley, chopped

2 eggs, lightly beaten
1 tsp cumin
Pinch of cayenne
Celtic salt and pepper
Vegetable oil

1. In a pan, roast the cumin seeds on the stove until they are fragrant. Grind in a spice mill.
2. In a mixing bowl, combine lamb, onion, garlic, parsley, eggs, cumin, cayenne pepper, salt and pepper.
3. Using your hands, shape the mixture into 1½-inch balls; flatten them slightly so they look more like rectangular cubes than spheres.
4. Depending on the length of your skewers, thread about 2-3 meatballs on each skewer. Rub or brush a little oil on the meat balls.
5. Cook on the grill about 5 minutes on each side, or until the meat is no longer showing a pink colour inside.
6. Serve immediately with a hot sauce, a salad and/or the **Grilled Vegetables Side Dish**☺ below.

☺**Grilled Vegetables Side Dish:** Since you have the grill hot, you might as well grill a few vegetables to go with the skewers. Cut the vegetables into bite-size pieces and combine in a mixing bowl.

Here are a few options:

- **Peppers,** red, orange, yellow and green, cut in quarters and seeded, grilled for 5-7 minutes. To make the peeling easier, place them in a paper bag and allow them to sweat for a few minutes.
- **Onions**, peeled and cut in quarters, grilled for 5-8 minutes.
- **Zucchini**, cut in thick slices, grilled until softened and juicy.

Add 3 chopped **tomatoes**, 1 cup **green or black olives**, 2 tbsp **capers**, fresh chopped **parsley**, **hot pepper flakes**, **lemon zest**, some **lemon juice**, a few glugs of **olive oil**, some **salt and pepper**. Toss and serve.

Grilled Surf & Turf

Serves 6-8
Prep Time: 15 min.
Marinating Time: 4 hours
Cooking Time: 20-30 min.

This is a great dish to serve for a casual summer gathering by the barbecue.
The marinade and the meats can be prepared up to a day in advance and kept in the refrigerator.
You can serve it with an assortment of grilled vegetables, and salads.

Marinade:

In a measuring cup, whisk the following ingredients:

¼ cup olive oil
¼ cup white wine vinegar
4-6 garlic cloves, minced
1 tbsp fresh rosemary, finely chopped

1 tbsp fresh oregano, finely chopped
1 tbsp fresh parsley, finely chopped
2 tsp hot red pepper, or to taste
Celtic salt and pepper

Meats:

8 lamb shops
8 chicken thighs, extra fat removed

16 large shrimp, shelled but tail still on, and deveined
4 chorizo or Italian sausages

1. Distribute the marinade into 3 bowls.
2. In the 1st bowl, add the lamb chops with the marinade, and toss to coat.
3. In the 2nd bowl, add the chicken thighs with the marinade, and toss to coat.
4. Do not add anything in the 3rd bowl yet, it will be for the shrimp later.
5. Cover all 3 bowls with some food wrap. Transfer the bowls to the refrigerator, and marinate for 4 hours or until the next day. (Yes, even the 3rd bowl is being marinated!)
6. Half an hour before grilling time, remove the bowls from the refrigerator. In the 3rd bowl, add the shrimp, toss to coat. Marinate for 30 minutes.
7. Meanwhile, start the barbecue and cook the sausages until they are no longer pink inside, about 25 minutes, rotating them so they cook on all sides. Transfer to a serving platter and keep warm.
8. Cook the lamb chops and the chicken thighs about 15 minutes, or until they are no longer pink inside, turning them over once.
9. Meanwhile, place the shrimp on the grill and cook about 5 minutes, until they turn pink, turning them over once. Transfer lamb, chicken and shrimp to the serving platter. Enjoy at once.

"Common sense is instinct, and enough of it is genius."
-Josh Billings, U.S. humorist

Swimming Protein with Scales and Shells

Fish and Seafood

Anyone born or having grown up near the sea has salt water coursing in his or her veins. They know fish and seafood, from the daily activities at the harbour, the "catch of the day" at the local fish store, the well-anticipated seasonal treats from the sea, to the fishermen's stories.

My ancestors' roots have been established along the seashores of Normandy, France and the St-Lawrence River in Québec. I feel happiest when I am near water where I can smell the salty air, listen to the waves and the birds, wait for the tide to go out so I can walk barefoot on the cold sand banks, and look at beautiful seashells and small creatures.
I see the ocean as a refreshing garden for inspiration and my favourite vacation destination.

I had my fair share of fish and seafood growing up on the St-Lawrence River in Québec, where my father and friends often went fishing and brought home many meals to enjoy in numerous ways: pan-fried, baked, poached, grilled, marinated, dried and salted, smoked. Up until 25-30 years, every year at the end of May and early June, a natural phenomenon used to take place on the shores of the St-Lawrence under the midnight moon. Millions of small fish, called *capelans*, literally "rolled" with the tide onto the shore where they could easily be scooped up by anyone who wanted some. One very early morning in June, while visiting my grandparents, I was caught snacking on some *capelans* that my great-grandfather had smoked and was drying inside the shed. Apparently, I was enjoying every bite, oblivious to the amused family elders who had gathered to watch me. I was 4 years old.

We often had (and still do) fish for breakfast, a menu choice not unusual in countries like Japan, China, and the Scandinavian regions. It was common knowledge that fish is food for the brain. We also consumed fish oils as a dietary supplement.

I find fresh fish and seafood the easiest food to prepare because not much is required to bring out their delicate flavour, sweetness, juicy-ness, and tender texture. Steaming, pan-frying, baking, grilling or poaching are often the quickest and most effective methods of cooking fish and seafood to guarantee the best flavours and to keep their glistening textures intact. Just a few minutes of cooking and basic flavouring – such as citrus juice and zest, herbs, spices, oil, some vegetables, and even fruits – are all that is required to make a fish or seafood dish simple but outstanding in flavours.

Whenever possible, for optimal taste and quality, when you shop at your favourite fish store, request fish and seafood fresh from the sea instead of a fish farm where they may have been fed antibiotics and other offensively toxic agents.

Sautéed Scallops with *Piment d'Espelette* and Lime Juice

Serves 2-4
Prep Time: 5 min.
Cooking Time: 10 min.

You can use large scallops or the smaller Bay scallops that will require less cooking time.
Piment d'Espelette is a variety of red pepper from the southwestern French
region of Espelette in the Pyrénées-Atlantiques.
It is sweet and mildly hot. In the Basque region, this spice is often used in place of black pepper.
If you can't find it, you can substitute it with ground hot pepper flakes.

1 lb of fresh scallops, cut in half so you have thin disks
Celtic salt and pepper
1 tsp ground *piment d'Espelette*
A handful of fresh chives or basil or coriander, finely chopped
Juice of 1 lime
2 tbsp olive oil

1. Rinse the scallops and pat dry. Season with salt, pepper and *piment d'Espelette*.
2. In a non-stick pan, add oil and cook the scallops over medium heat, until they are golden, constantly turning them. Pour the lime juice in the pan while you continue to stir the scallops. Garnish with the chopped chives and serve immediately.

Thai Steamed Fish

Serves 4
Prep Time: 15-20 min.
Steaming Time: 18-20 min.

You can use any fresh fish available in your area. If the fish is too small for 4 servings, you may want to buy 2 and double the quantity of the seasoning. Or you can use large fish pieces. The sauce becomes fragrant and mouth-watering during the steaming process.
No fish steamer? No worries! You can improvise one by using a baking dish large enough to hold the fish, and placing a rack on the bottom. **No rack?** No problem! You can improvise one, too! Scrub and cut lengthwise a few large carrots and celery stalks onto which the fish will rest above the steaming water.

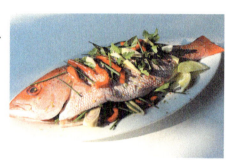

1 whole red snapper of 3-4 lbs, cleaned, scaled
1 piece of fresh gingerroot of about 1 inch, peeled, sliced thinly
2 garlic cloves, peeled and thinly sliced
1 tbsp each of fresh basil and coriander leaves
3 green onions, cut into 2-inch pieces, or a handful of chives
1 red sweet pepper, cut into thin strips
1 lemongrass stem, cut into 1-inch pieces

Sauce:

In a bowl, combine together: ¼ cup organic Tamari,
2 tbsp sucanat or cane sugar, the juice of 1 lime,
2 tsp sesame oil, and a pinch of red pepper flakes

Garnish:

Lime wedges

1. Make 4 diagonal slits on one side of the fish, spacing them equally and cutting to the backbone. Insert 1 slice of ginger, 1 slice of garlic, 1 basil leaf and 1 cilantro leaf into each slit. Turn fish over. Make 4 diagonal slits and insert remaining slices of ginger, garlic, basil and cilantro leaves. Place fish in a fish steamer.
2. Sprinkle the sauce over the fish. Scatter the remaining ingredients over the fish and in the cavity near the backbone. Pour enough boiling water in the bottom of the steamer (real or improvised) to reach the bottom rack without touching the fish. Cover tightly with a lid or foil. Steam on top of the stove if using a steamer (or in the oven at 350°F if using a baking dish) until the fish is just flaky, but not dry, about 18-20 minutes. Serve with lime wedges and the fish juices.

Thai Curried Shrimp

Serves 4
Prep Time: 15-20 min.
Cooking Time: 15-20 min.

You can enjoy it as a stew over chunks of boiled sweet potatoes.

Zest and juice of 2 oranges, reserve the juice
1 lb large shrimp, peeled and deveined
1 tbsp curry powder
Celtic salt and pepper
1 tbsp olive oil + 1 tbsp olive oil
1 small onion, diced
1 green pepper, chopped
1 red pepper, chopped

1½ cups frozen or fresh peas
A large handful of green beans, trimmed and cut in half
½ zucchini, chopped
2 kaffir lime leaves
1 cup tomato juice
1 can coconut milk
10 basil leaves, chopped
Basil leaves to garnish

1. In a large bowl, combine half of the zest with the shrimp, 1½ tsp curry powder, salt and pepper. Toss to coat.
2. Heat 1 tbsp oil in a large skillet over medium heat. Cook shrimp until bright pink, about 2 minutes per side. Transfer to a plate.
3. Heat remaining tablespoon of oil. Add onion, vegetables, and remaining 1½ tsp curry powder. Cook until the onion is translucent, about 4 minutes. Add kaffir lime leaves, orange and tomato juices; cook until liquid starts to thicken, about 6-8 minutes.
4. Return the shrimp to the skillet, and cook until heated through, about 2 minutes. Stir in the coconut milk. Add remaining orange zest; season with salt and pepper. Serve garnished with basil leaves over boiled sweet potato chunks.

*"I will keep my dignity and self-respect, as well as yours;
therefore, I will not lower myself to insult or speak ill of you."*
--Unknown

Spanish Shrimp and Tomatoes

Serves 4
Prep Time: 10-15 min.
Cooking Time: 12-15 min.

Three words that will make you love it: easy, quick, flavourful!
You can serve it with a salad or over steamed spinach.

1 tbsp olive or coconut oil
1½ lbs shrimp, peeled, deveined
Celtic salt and pepper
2 garlic cloves, thinly sliced
Hot pepper flakes
A few strands of saffron, diluted in ¼ cup of warm water
6 plum tomatoes, cored, halved lengthwise, and sliced in ½-inch thick
2 tbsp each chopped parsley and basil
1 tbsp each of lemon and orange juice and some of their zest
¼ cup pine nuts or almond slivers, lightly toasted

1. In a large non-stick skillet, heat the oil over medium-high heat. Swirl to coat the skillet. Season the shrimp. Add half the shrimp to the skillet and cook until opaque and pink through, 3-4 minutes. Transfer to a plate. Repeat with the remaining shrimp, adding more oil if necessary.
2. Reduce heat to medium. Add garlic and pepper flakes. Stir in the saffron water and the tomatoes. Cook until the tomatoes begin to break down, 4-6 minutes. Season with salt.
3. Return the shrimp and any accumulated juices to the skillet. Add parsley, basil, lemon and orange juice and their zest. Toss to coat. Sprinkle the pine nuts or almonds.

Do you know what 'aristology' is?
It is the art of dining well

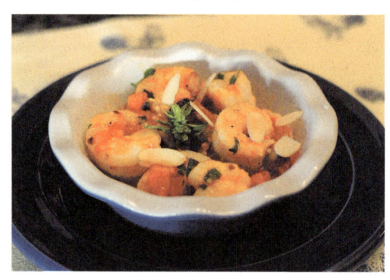

Satisfying the Sweet Tooth

Desserts

Did you know that "STRESSED" is "DESSERTS" spelled backward?
Doesn't a little dessert make you feel better when you are stressed, tired and need a little comfort?
There are special occasions that require decadent desserts, and,
without a beautiful mouth-watering dessert, the celebration wouldn't be complete, right?
Desserts are fun to make and even more fun to eat. After all, desserts make people very happy!

In moderation, the healthier fruit-based, spice-flavored spa indulgences in this chapter
will help you "reset" yourself without feeling guilty, remorseful, or ill afterwards.
Or having to run a 10K marathon to burn off the excess calories!

I don't have dessert often. But, when I do, it has to be pretty spectacular by my books.
Desserts made with seasonal ripe fruits at the peak of their perfection, are by far my favourite:
they are quick to make, they are fresh, juicy-sweet, and brightly colored.
They are full of tasty vitamins; therefore, a healthier option. I never feel that I am sacrificing taste and pleasure.

To help prevent overeating (and ingesting unwanted extra calories),
knowing that there is a delicious dessert waiting for you at the end of dinner,
allow yourself to stop eating long before you feel full and uncomfortable so you can enjoy the sweet treat guilt-free.
And don't eat again until breakfast the next day.

I hope you, too, will find that the following recipes for occasional treats can satisfy your craving for sweets
without making you overeat, feel stuffed and regretful afterwards. Enjoy and feel good!

Below: *A rainbow of fresh fruits: strawberries, blood oranges, fuyu persimmons, pineapple,
kiwis, blueberries, blackberries and cherries. Pretty, juicy and simple.*

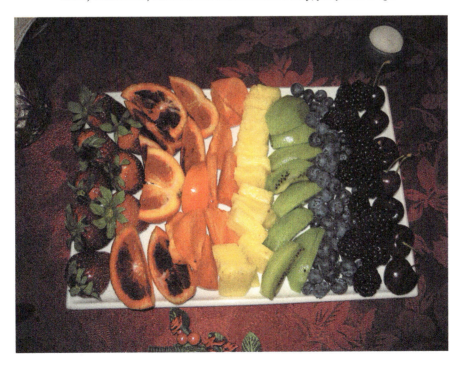

1-Vibrant Fruit Desserts

Pineapple with Mint Paste

Serves 4-6
Prep Time: 15 min.

This is an amazingly cooling treat that you and your family will savour and polish off quickly. Guaranteed! The bright green of the mint against the golden yellow of the pineapple makes this fruit dessert so irresistible. A great festive light dessert that is perfect for the Holiday season.

1 fresh pineapple, peeled, cored and cut into chunks or in thin half-moons
2 cups of fresh mint leaves
2-4 tbsp cane sugar or sucanat or coconut sugar
To garnish: Lime zest, pomegranate seeds, and extra mint leaves

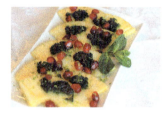

1. Arrange the pineapple chunks or half-moons on a serving platter.
2. With a pestle and mortar, bruise and crush the mint leaves with the sugar or sucanat, working the mass into a paste. Add more sugar if needed to achieve a moist, bright green paste.
3. With a spatula or a spoon, spread the paste over the pineapple pieces.
4. **To garnish:** Sprinkle the lime zest and the pomegranate seeds on top. Garnish with mint leaves.

Peaches Cardinal

Serves 4
Prep Time: 15-20 min.
Cooking Time: 2 min.
Chilling Time: a few hours

So delicious when the peaches and the raspberries are in season!

2½ cups fresh raspberries
2 tsp cane sugar or sucanat or coconut sugar

4 large ripe peaches or nectarines (yellow or white flesh)
Fresh mint sprig for garnishing

1. Put the raspberries in a food processor or blender and whirl until puréed. To remove the seeds, using a spatula, press the mixture through a fine sieve resting over a bowl. Discard the seeds.
2. Add the sugar or sucanat to the puréed raspberries and stir in.
3. Bring a pot of water to a boil. With a knife, carve an X on the bottom of each peach. Place the peaches in the hot water and leave for 1 minute. Remove from the water and carefully peel the skin.
4. Allow the peaches to cool; then, cut them in half and remove the stone. Put 2 halves in each serving glass.
5. Drizzle the purée over the peaches, cover and chill for a few hours. Serve garnished with mint leaves.

Note: If you are using fresh nectarines, you don't need to do Step 3: removing the peel.

Japanese Lychees and Melon Salad

Serves 4
Prep Time: 15 min.
Cooking Time: 8-10 min.
Chilling Time: 2-3 hours

A simple and elegant dessert. The syrup can be made ahead of time. At serving time, you can keep the vanilla bean pieces in the syrup or remove them. Native to China, the shiso leaf, or perilla or Japanese basil, has distinctive flavour notes of basil, mint and citrus. It is often used fresh in sushi rolls and rice dishes. It can be found in Asian markets, especially the Korean-Japanese grocery stores. Use fresh mint leaves if you can't find shiso leaves.

½ tsp each of lemon and lime zest
½ vanilla bean, thinly sliced
2 tbsp honey
3-4 cups of watermelon, peeled, seeded and cut into cubes

2 cups fresh lychees, peeled, seeded (or 1 can of lychees)
Seeds of ½ pomegranate
Shiso leaves or mint leaves, finely sliced with scissors

1. In a small saucepan, over high heat, combine zest, vanilla bean, honey and ¾ cup water. Stir until the honey has dissolved.
2. Bring to a boil; then, reduce the heat and simmer for 8-10 minutes to obtain a thin syrupy consistency.
3. Remove from the heat and allow to cool completely.
4. In a mixing bowl, gently toss the watermelon cubes and the lychees. Pour the chilled syrup over the fruits. Chill for 2-3 hours, gently toss once in a while.
5. To serve, sprinkle pomegranate seeds over the chilled fruits. Garnish with shiso or mint leaves.

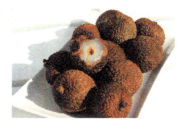

Strawberries with Balsamic Vinegar

Serves 4
Prep Time: 10 min.
Macerating Time: 2½ hours

A simple classic!

1 lb of ripe strawberries
¼ cup coconut sugar
2 tbsp balsamic vinegar
½ cup mascarpone cheese or whipped cream
Basil leaves, finely sliced with scissors

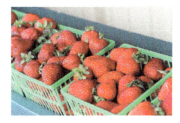

1. Wash the strawberries and wipe them dry. Remove the stems. Cut the big strawberries in half.
2. Place the strawberries in a large glass bowl, sprinkle the sugar over the top and toss gently to coat. Set aside for 2 hours to macerate. (They should be refrigerated if they will macerate for a longer period of time.)
3. Drizzle the balsamic vinegar over the strawberries. Toss again; then, refrigerate for ½ hour.
4. Spoon the strawberries into 4 glasses. Pour the syrup over them and top with a dollop of mascarpone or whipped cream. Garnish with the basil leaves.

Fraises au poivre noir
(Strawberries with black pepper)

Serves 4
Prep Time: 10 min.

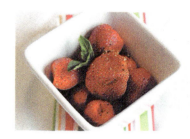

You may think that this is an unusual combination of flavours. You are right. Surprisingly, it tastes great! If you have to create a dessert in a hurry, this easy, no-bake fruit dessert can be put together in a flash. You can serve it with a small dollop of whipped cream. Anything is great with some whipped cream! Don't you agree?

3 cups of fresh strawberries
3 tbsp of sucanat or coconut sugar
2 tsp cracked black pepper

½ tsp orange zest
1 tbsp orange juice

Optional topping:

½ cup whipping cream and 1 tbsp sucanat or coconut sugar

1. Wash the strawberries and remove the stem.
2. Wrap them in paper towel to dry. You can cut them in half or leave them whole.
3. Put the strawberries in a bowl; add the sugar, the pepper, the orange zest and juice.
4. Allow to marinate for 5 minutes. While you wait, you have time to whip the cream with the sugar if you are using the topping.
5. Serve the strawberries with their juices and a spoonful of whipped cream. You can garnish with a few grains of pepper and a short strip of orange peel.

Grapes with Ginger, Lime and Mint

Serves 2-4
Prep Time: 5-10 min.

You will like this simple dessert for the refreshing flavours and just the right sweetness. You can also make this fruit salad a part of your breakfast.

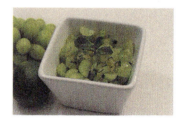

1 large bunch of seedless grapes (red, green or blue), about 3 cups
1-2 pieces of candied ginger, finely chopped
Zest of 1 lime

Juice of ½ lime
2 tbsp freshly chopped mint leaves
Mint leaves to garnish

1. Cut grapes in half and place in a salad bowl.
2. Add ginger, lime zest and juice, mint. Toss to combine.
3. Set aside for ½ hour. Garnish with mint leaves.

Variations:

- If the grapes are not very sweet, you can add 1 tbsp of honey.
- You can omit the lime juice and enjoy the concentrated lime essence of the zest.
- In place of candied ginger, you can grate 1½ tsp of fresh gingerroot.

Cantaloupe and Figs with Honey and Blue Cheese

Serves 4
Prep Time: 10 min.

This is a very quick and easy cheese course or dessert to put together. With the best ingredients that you can find, you can compose a beautiful and delicious platter of sweet and salty-pungent elements.

- 8-12 fresh Black Mission figs, halved
- 1 cantaloupe, cut into thin wedges
- 4-8 slices of blue cheese of your choice
- 2 tbsp almond slivers, toasted
- Honey for drizzling

On a serving platter, arrange the fig halves, the cantaloupe wedges, and the cheese slices. Sprinkle with the almonds, and drizzle with honey. Serve at room temperature.

Variation:

You can use honeydew wedges and fresh green figs, or mix and match the fruits for a different colour effect.

> *"Humor is the shock absorber of life; it helps us take the blows."*
> -Peggy Noonan, U.S. author

Mediterranean Date and Orange Salad

Serves 4
Prep Time: 15 min.
Simmering Time: 10 min.

The simple and easy-to-find ingredients allow you to make this salad any time of the year. Its spicy sweetness is quite warming and satisfying, especially on a cold day.

- 4 large oranges
- ⅓ cup dried apricots, halved
- 2 tbsp blanched almonds, toasted
- 2 tbsp fresh mint, chopped

Syrup:

- 1 cup water
- 2 star anise
- 1 cinnamon stick
- 6 cloves
- 1-2 tbsp honey
- ½ cup dried figs, sliced
- ½ cup seedless dates, halved

Cut both ends of the oranges. Cut the peel around the flesh, exposing the segments; then, over a bowl to collect the juices, carefully slice on both sides of each membrane and release the "naked" segments into the bowl. To the orange segments, add the apricots, almonds and mint. Add the syrup and mix well. You can enjoy this salad while the syrup is still warm or cooled.

Syrup:

Combine water, star anise, cinnamon, cloves and honey in a small saucepan. Simmer, uncovered, about 10 minutes or until thickened and slightly syrupy. Add the figs and dates. Allow to cool for a few minutes. Discard the star anise, the cinnamon stick and the cloves.

Red Grapefruit and Pomegranate Salad

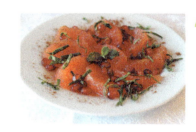

Serves 4
Prep Time: 5-10 min.
Cooking Time: 5 min.
Chilling Time: 15 min.

Very fragrant and refreshing, this fresh fruit salad is perfect when you want a light dessert after a copious meal. The rose water fragrance gives this salad an exotic tone. If possible, choose red and white grapefruits for an appealing colour contrast.

4 red grapefruits, or pomello, peeled and cut into skinless segments or *suprêmes*
Seeds from 1 pomegranate
1-2 tbsp honey

1 tsp rose water
Ground cinnamon
4-5 fresh mint leaves, finely cut with scissors

1. In a small saucepan, warm the honey in 4 tbsp of water. Allow to cool for about 15 minutes. Add the rose water.
2. **To serve,** on a platter or individual plates, arrange each grapefruit segment around the platter, pointing to the centre. Sprinkle the pomegranate seeds over the segments. Drizzle the honey sauce over the salad and sprinkle with some cinnamon. Scatter the finely cut mint leaves over the top.

Trois fondues au chocolat

Serves 4-6
Prep Time : 20-30 min.
Warming Time: 5-10 min.

These chocolate fondues are decadent, sinful and sooo goood! Spa food doesn't have to be blah food. Because they have an incredible amount of antioxidants, fruit and chocolate are very good for you. This is quite an interactive dessert to share leisurely with a group of guests after a good dinner. I love serving it outdoors on a warm summer evening when the guests are not in a rush to go back home and they just want to enjoy the food, folks and fun in the glow of candlelight and fondue tea lights. Choose the recipe that appeals to you, or make more than one to give your guests exponential pleasure!

Recipe #1 French Almond Fondue

1 lb Toblerone chocolate, cut in pieces
¼ lb semisweet chocolate, cut in pieces
½ cup 35% cream

½ cup toasted almonds, chopped
6 tbsp kirsch or Framboise (a raspberry liqueur)

Recipe #2 Spanish Orange Fondue

6 oz of dark chocolate, coarsely chopped
2 oz milk chocolate, coarsely chopped
¼ cup heavy cream
½ tsp vanilla
1 tsp ground cinnamon

Pinch of Celtic salt
Pinch of cayenne pepper or hot red pepper flakes
2 tbsp Triple Sec or Grand Marnier
Finely grated orange zest and juice

Recipe #3 White Chocolate Fondue

⅓ cup heavy cream
1 tbsp of peach or pear schnapps (optional)

Very finely grated zest of 1 lemon, or more
8 squares (8 oz) best-quality white chocolate, chopped

Dippers: Cut in chunks, slices or cubes an assortment of fresh exotic fruits such as kiwis, oranges, cantaloupe, honeydew, strawberries, starfruit, pineapple, mandarin oranges, seedless grapes, cherries, lychees, slices of banana, apple and pear brushed with some lemon juice to prevent browning. You can also add pieces of dried fruit like pear, apricot or mango.

Important Notes for all Three Recipes:

The chocolate will coat the fruit dippers more easily if they have been chilled. Arrange all fresh fruit pieces on a nice serving platter and garnish with some mint leaves or sprigs. Provide fondue forks or long wooden sticks to spear the fruit pieces and dip in the melted chocolate mixture. If you don't have a chocolate fondue pot, use a regular fondue pot. Remember that chocolate dessert fondues should not boil as it will impair the flavour. Also, chocolate burns very easily.

Recipe #1

In a saucepan, over low heat, melt the 2 chocolates. Add the cream, the almonds and the liqueur. Once all combined, pour in a chocolate fondue pot and keep warm over a lit tea light.

Recipe #2

In a saucepan, over low heat, combine the two chocolates and cream, stirring frequently until the mixture is creamy and the chocolates have completely melted. Add the rest of the ingredients and stir to combine. If the mixture is too thick, stir in a couple of tablespoons of cream as needed to create a good dipping consistency. Pour in a chocolate fondue pot and keep warm over a lit tea light.

Recipe #3

In the top part of a double boiler (or *bain-Marie*: cooking in a pot or bowl that is partially immersed in hot water), set over simmering water, heat gently the cream, schnapps, and lemon zest. Add the chocolate and stir until smooth. Please note that white chocolate is very thin when hot. If you prefer a thicker fondue, turn off the burner, let cool and chill for 1-2 hours before serving.

Poached Peaches

Serves 4
Prep Time: 10-15 min.
Cooking Time: 1 hour

Any stone fruit would be great in this recipe, either a single variety or a combination like plums, nectarines and apricots. A poaching fruit dessert is a no-fail, very easy dessert option, especially if baking is not your strength. The poaching can be done ahead of time, even days ahead. It is an ideal method to transform slightly under-ripe fruit, or fruit that don't look as appealing into fork-tender, highly flavourful delicacies. So, go ahead and give it a try.

4 cups water
¼ cup coconut sugar or another sweetener
1 vanilla bean, split and scraped
6 cardamom pods
3 star anise pods
1 cinnamon stick

4 peaches, halved and pitted
Freshly whipped cream (optional)
Fresh mint sprigs

1. In a saucepan that can hold all 8 peach halves, bring to a simmer the water, sugar, vanilla bean and seeds, and spices. Stir until the sugar has dissolved.
2. Add the peach halves and push them down so they are submerged. Cover, and simmer until the fruit are just fork-tender, about 6-8 minutes. With a slotted spoon, transfer the fruit to a dish. Cover them with foil.
3. Bring the poaching liquid to a boil, and cook until it is reduced to about 1½ cups, about 40 minutes. Strain and discard the spices: they have fulfilled their purpose.
4. Let the reduced liquid (a fragrant syrupy nectar at this point) cool. Serve the peach halves in pretty bowls, and spoon the liquid over. If you wish, to complete the decadence, add a small spoonful of whipped cream and garnish with mint leaves.

Roasted Grapes with Mascarpone Cream

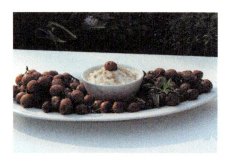

Serves 4
Prep Time: 15-20 min.
Roasting Time: 15 min.

1 lb seedless grapes, red or purple or a combination, left on the stems and cut into small clusters
2 tsp honey
1 tbsp orange juice

1 tsp each of orange zest and olive oil
½ tsp Celtic salt
¼ tsp each of ground cinnamon, clove, and ginger

Mascarpone Cream:

½ cup mascarpone
1 tsp vanilla

2 tsp honey or maple syrup
Zest of ½ an orange and its juice

1. Preheat the oven to 475°F. In a large mixing bowl, gently toss the grape clusters, honey, orange juice and zest, oil, salt and spices. Spread the grapes in a single layer on a large rimmed baking sheet. Roast for about 15 minutes, flipping halfway through, until they are collapsed, juicy, fragrant, and beginning to caramelize.
2. While the grapes are roasting, prepare the cream. In a small mixing bowl, stir together the mascarpone, vanilla, honey, zest and juice. Transfer the roasted grapes to serving dishes, and serve warm with a dollop of the flavoured mascarpone cream.

Thai Tropical Fruit Salad with a Papaya Sauce

Serves 4
Prep Time: 20 min.

Salad:

1 mango
¼ pineapple
16-20 lychees (you can also use rambutans and/or longans)

2 kiwis
½ pomello
1 banana

Sauce:

1 ripe papaya peeled, seeded, and roughly chopped
Finely grated zest and juice of 1 lime
½ cup pineapple juice or another tropical fruit juice
To garnish: kaffir lime leaves or mint leaves

Salad:

Prepare an assortment of tropical fruits and cut them into bite-size pieces. Place them in serving bowl.

Sauce:

Place the papaya chunks in a food processor with ¾ of the lime zest and its juice. Add the pineapple juice or tropical fruit juice. Purée until smooth, and add more juice if it is too thick. Taste and add more lime juice if desired.

Assembly:

Serve the fruit salad in pretty bowls. Spoon some of the sauce over and scatter the remaining lime zest over the top. Garnish each salad with a kaffir lime leaf or mint leaf.

Indian-spiced Fruit in an Almond Milk Bath

Serves 4-6
Prep Time: 10-15 min.
Cooking Time: 5-10 min.

Very colourful and healthy, this dessert will please everyone.

⅓ cup sliced almonds
2 cups unsweetened almond milk
(or any other milk you like)
1 tbsp honey (or more if you want a sweeter taste)
½ tsp ground cardamom
Pinch of saffron
¾ cup fresh fruit, prepared and cut in small pieces, like lychees, mango, papaya, pineapple, banana
To garnish: shelled pistachios, pomegranate seeds, chopped mint leaves

1. Place the almonds and the milk in a blender; whirl until smooth.
2. In a saucepan, heat and stir the almond mixture to a boil. Remove from heat; stir in honey, cardamom, saffron and fruit pieces. Transfer to a serving bowl. Refrigerate until serving time. Garnish with pistachios, pomegranate seeds and chopped mint.

Did you know that India contributed the most number of original spices to the art of cooking?

Italian Panna Cotta

Serves 6-8
Prep Time: 30 min.
Cooking Time: 15 min.
Chilling Time: at least 3 hours

This cool dessert can be topped with fresh berries, a fruit coulis, even flaxseeds flavoured with cinnamon. Served in pretty glassware, it will impress and refresh your guests.

6 tbsp cold water
2 envelopes of unflavoured gelatin
2 cups of heavy cream or full-fat coconut milk from a can
½ cup honey
1 tbsp pure vanilla extract
To garnish: fresh berries or fresh cut fruit; fresh mint leaves

1. In a large mixing bowl, pour the water and sprinkle the gelatin over the top. Let it do its magic for 10 minutes or so.
2. In a saucepan, add the cream or milk, and cook over medium heat until hot but not to the boiling point. Remove the saucepan from the heat, and add the honey and the vanilla. Stir well to dissolve the honey. Cool for a few minutes.
3. Pour the warm mixture over the gelatin, and gently whisk until the gelatin is completely dissolved.
4. Pour the liquid into dessert cups or regular glasses. Refrigerate for at least 3 hours, until the Panna Cotta is set and firm.
5. Garnish with fresh berries or fruits, and mint leaves.

Variation:

For a Mediterranean flavour, while the cream or milk is being heated in step 2, you can add a pinch of saffron threads, 8 crushed cardamom pods, and 2 cinnamon sticks. In step 3, using a strainer, pour the warm mixture over the gelatin. Continue with the rest of the recipe.

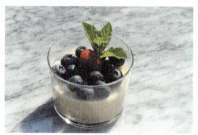

Spanish-inspired "Chocolado" Pudding-like Mousse

(I know; it is quite a mouthful! But wait until you try a mouthful of this velvety delight!)

Serves 4
Prep Time: 10 min.
Cooling Time: 1 hour or more

This delicious avocado-based treat will satisfy any craving for sweets. No baking, no dairy, no fuss! So, what do you get beside a mouth-watering dessert? Fiber (from the medjool dates), a boost for the metabolism, lots of antioxidants, and the virtuous feeling that you are actually indulging in something wholesome and awesome!

2 ripe avocados
⅓ cup of honey
2 medjool dates, pitted
½ cup cocoa
1 tsp vanilla

Pinch of cayenne pepper and cinnamon
Pinch of Celtic salt
Almond milk (to thin the mousse, as needed)
To garnish: fresh fruit and mint leaves

1. Combine all ingredients in a blender or food processor until smooth, scraping down the sides with a spatula. While the machine is running, add as much almond milk, in small amounts, as you want to thin the mousse to reach the desired texture and thickness.
2. Pour in pretty glass containers and refrigerate until serving time. You can garnish with fresh fruit and mint leaves.

Flavoured Whipped Cream

Of all the wonderful toppings for any dessert, this is my favourite finishing touch. Everybody loves real whipped cream: it is so simple but decadent. It beats by several miles the store-bought canned version. If you are going to treat yourself to a dessert, make sure it is a satisfying one with the best ingredients. This way, you will thoroughly enjoy it and feel happy, instead of *wishing* it was the real thing and compensate by eating more of the not-so-good second choice.
Just a spoonful will do! Remember – moderation!

Here are a few ideas to jazz it up.

1. **Basic Recipe:** In a cold, deep bowl, pour 2 cups of 35% **whipping cream**. Place the bowl in the sink to prevent the splashes from going everywhere: it saves on the clean-up effort and time! With an electric beater, or by

hand with a whisk (if you don't already have strong arm muscles, you will develop some while whipping!), whip the cream on medium speed for a few minutes.

   Flavouring: When it is gradually thickening, add 1-2 tbsp of **sweetener like maple syrup,** and 1 tsp **vanilla extract**. Increase the power and whip until firm peaks form. (Don't beat too long or you will get vanilla butter! Not a total waste, it can be used in a cake. But it is not what you want here.) Depending on the dessert you want to serve the cream with, you can also add **orange** or **lime zest**, and **spices like cinnamon** that you combine very gently into the cream. Refrigerate until serving time.

2. **Chocolate whipped cream:** Sift 2-3 tbsp **unsweetened cocoa**. Add to the cream and follow the directions for the Basic Recipe. Add 1-2 tbsp **maple syrup**, and beat until firm peaks form. This mixture is ideal for icing a cake.
3. **Honey and yogurt:** Whip together ¼ cup **plain Greek yogurt**, ⅔ cup of 35% **whipping cream**, and 2 tbsp **liquid honey** until firm peaks form. Great on crêpes or over fresh fruit.

"My heart is in the right place.
I know, because I hid it there."
-Carrie Fisher, actor, screenwriter, novelist

2-Wholesome and Nourishing Baking

Breads, Crackers, Muffins and Cookies

"Paleotizing" my favourite baked recipes has required researching for non-offensive ingredients and creative tweaking. I know that it is possible to create food that is delicious and exciting.

I am the first to admit that nothing bakes as well and tastes as good as wheat flour!

However, I feel so much better after eating my "new and improved" occasional treats made with healthier and more wholesome ingredients.
And I certainly don't miss the *addictive* aspect and side effects of wheat-based baked goods.

The following recipes for easily baked goods don't depend on exact measuring and skilled hands to be delicious and successfully achieved, but rather on *fresh* ingredients and *a relaxed approach*.

So, relax and have fun with the following recipes, and experiment on your own.
You can't muff it up!

I hope you will enjoy these recipes and find that there is life without wheat and gluten and that, in fact, it is an even better life.

Mediterranean Herb Loaf

Makes 10-12 slices
Prep Time: 20 min.
Cooking Time: 65-75 min.
Cooling Time: 40 min.

I found a similar recipe in a gluten-free baking book and tweaked the ingredients to Philip's preference.
The sweet variation with cinnamon and raisins was his request.
The delicate slices are great with a spread, savory or sweet.
They also make great toasts; it is best to toast them horizontally in the toaster oven.

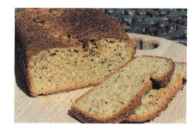

2 cups ground almonds
1 cup ground flaxseeds, golden or brown
2 tsp baking powder
1 tsp xantham gum
1 tsp Celtic salt
½ tsp each of dried parsley, basil, oregano, rosemary
1 tbsp fresh chives, finely cut with scissors

½ tsp hot pepper flakes
1 tbsp dehydrated onion flakes
4-5 eggs
1 cup unsweetened almond milk
1 tbsp maple syrup
½ cup melted butter

1. Preheat the oven to 375°F. Prepare a baking loaf pan by lining it with a piece of parchment paper that is lightly oiled or buttered.
2. In a medium bowl, combine the almonds, flaxseeds, baking powder, xantham gum, salt, herbs, hot pepper flakes and dehydrated onion flakes. Whisk until well combined.
3. In a larger bowl, whisk or mix together with a hand-held mixer the eggs, milk, maple syrup and butter until homogeneous.
4. In batches, add the dry ingredients to the egg mixture and mix with a spoon or a hand-held mixer for 1-2 minutes to make a smooth, sticky but easy to spread batter.

5. Pour the mixture into the prepared pan, leveling the top. Bake for 35 minutes. Rotate and bake for 30-35 minutes more, until golden brown and the top has risen and is springy when pressed in the centre. A toothpick inserted in the centre should come out clean.
6. Let the loaf cool in the pan for 10 minutes or more. Lift the loaf out of the pan using the parchment paper. Let it cool on a cooling rack for 30 minutes or so before slicing and serving it. The loaf will deflate a little during the cooling period.

Variations:

- Instead of almond milk, you can use cow's milk.
- You can vary the herbs. You can add toasted pine nuts, chopped kalamata olives, and finely sliced sun-dried tomatoes with the dry ingredients. Adding some grated parmesan makes the loaf fragrant and tasty.
- Instead of a savory loaf, you can make a dessert bread by substituting the herbs, hot pepper flakes and dried onion flakes with ground spices like cinnamon, nutmeg, clove, ginger; adding ⅓ cup of raisins, and using 2 tbsp of maple syrup instead of one.

Breakfast Almond Buns

Serves 4-6
Prep Time: 15-20 min.
Cooking Time: 25-30 min.

Here is another option for a grain-free bread. Need another breakfast idea? When sliced, the bottom half of the bun can be the bed onto which you rest a few slices of cooked bacon and a beautifully poached or over-easy cooked egg. All you have to do is enjoy. And decide what you want to do with the top half!

1 cup blanched almond flour	¼ cup cold butter, cut in cubes
2 tbsp flaxseeds	1 egg, at room temperature
1 tsp baking powder	2 tbsp unsweetened almond milk
½ tsp Celtic salt	2 egg whites, at room temperature
¼ tsp pepper	

1. Preheat the oven to 350°F. Line a baking sheet with parchment paper. Set aside.
2. In a mixing bowl, whisk together almond flour, flaxseeds, baking powder, salt and pepper.
3. With a fork or your fingers, incorporate the butter into the flour mixture until you obtain pea-size crumbs. Add the whole egg and milk; mix with a fork to combine.
4. In a separate bowl, whip egg whites until stiff peaks form. Gently fold the egg whites into the bun batter until fully combined.
5. Drop about 2 tbsp of batter per bun on the baking sheet. Bake for 25-30 minutes.
6. Let the buns cool for 5 minutes. Remove from baking sheet and carefully slice in half.

Variations:

- Instead of 1 cup of blanched ground almond flour, use only ¾ cup, and add ¼ cup ground walnut flour.
- Use fresh herbs like parsley
- Add ½ tsp of various spices like caraway seeds or aniseeds.

*"I burned 60 calories.
That should take care of the peanut I had in 1962."*
--Rita Rudner, actress

Asian Crackers

Makes about 50 crackers
Prep Time: 15 min.
Cooking Time: 12-15 min.

These crackers can be enjoyed plain or topped with an interesting spread like tapenade, salmon mousse, guacamole, etc.
They make a great snack on the go. You can also freeze half the dough to be used later.

A- Dry ingredients

3 cups almond flour
1½ tsp Celtic salt
½ cup natural almonds, finely chopped or ⅓ cup hazelnut flour or a combination of the two

1 tbsp sesame seeds, lightly toasted
1 tsp garlic powder or onion flakes

B- Wet ingredients

1 tbsp + 1 tsp coconut oil, melted
1 tsp sesame oil
1 tsp ginger, finely grated

2 eggs
1 tsp lime zest
1 tbsp chives, finely cut with scissors

1. Preheat the oven to 350°F. Prepare 2 large baking sheets by lining them with a piece of parchment each. Cut a 3rd piece of the same size. Set aside.
2. In a large bowl, combine the ingredients in the **A** section.
3. In another bowl, whisk the **B** ingredients.
4. Stir the wet **B** ingredients into the dry **A** mixture until well combined.
5. Divide the dough into 2 pieces. Place 1 piece of dough between 2 sheets of parchment paper and, with a rolling pin, roll from the centre outwards until the dough is about 1/16-inch thick.
6. Remove the top piece of parchment paper and transfer the bottom piece of parchment with the rolled-out dough onto a baking sheet. Repeat the process with the remaining piece of dough.
7. Trim the excess dough off the sides to create straight edges and roll out the trimmed parts again. Cut the dough into 2-inch squares with a knife or pizza cutter.
8. Bake for 12-15 minutes, until lightly golden. Let the crackers cool on the baking sheets for 30 minutes before serving.

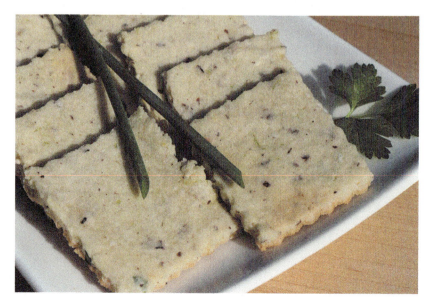

Bananapple Muffins with Spices

Makes 14-16
Prep Time: 20 min.
Cooking Time: 18-20 min.

A-1 ripe banana, mashed with a fork
4 eggs, lightly beaten
1 tsp vanilla
2 tbsp maple syrup
⅓ cup water
1 apple, finely grated

B-2 cup ground almond meal
¼ cup ground flaxseeds
½ tsp baking soda
½ tsp baking powder
1 tsp ground cinnamon
½ tsp ground cloves
¼ tsp ground ginger
¼ tsp ground nutmeg
½ tsp Celtic salt

C-¼ cup melted coconut oil

1. Preheat the oven to 350°F. Prepare a muffin tin by lining the holes with paper muffin cups. Or lightly grease the tin with melted coconut oil.
2. In a large mixing bowl, combine the **A** ingredients.
3. In a smaller bowl, whisk the dry **B** ingredients together.
4. Pour the melted oil (**C**) in the wet banana mixture and whisk together.
5. Pour half the dry ingredients into the wet ingredients; mix with a wooden spoon. Add the rest of the dry ingredients and mix until combined.
6. Fill each muffin hole ¾ of the way to the top, leaving room for expansion. Dust a little ground cinnamon on top of muffins. Bake 18-20 minutes or until a toothpick inserted in the middle of a muffin comes out clean. Serve while hot.

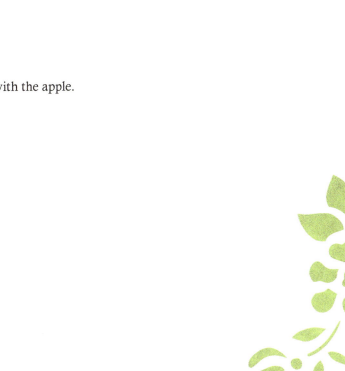

Variations:

- Instead of an apple, you can use a ripe pear.
- You can create a different spice combination.
- Finely chopped candied ginger and raisins are great with the apple.

Gratitude

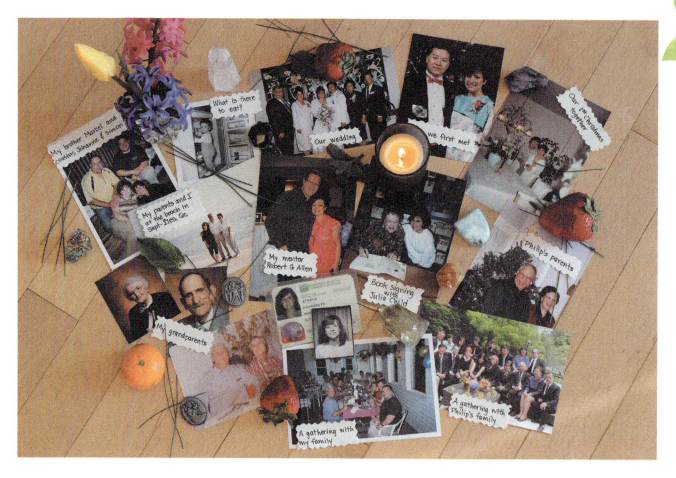

"No matter what accomplishments you achieve, somebody helped you."
--Althea Gibson

"The only people with whom you should try to get even are those who have helped you."
-May Maloo, writer

I couldn't have created this nourishment book without the support, the encouragement, and the spiritual and emotional *nourishment* from the people who held the space for me and this project. The loving support and assistance I received from you made me feel like I was carried on a magical carpet to complete this journey; and because of your supporting presence and encouraging words, I could not NOT have reached my destination! I owe all of you my most heart-felt gratitude.

Philip, *l'amour de ma vie*, my precious husband and life partner, for always being next to me for yet another BIG project! I wouldn't be able to successfully accomplish as much with most of my sanity intact without your unwavering assistance, your steady fire energy and your loving patience. Besides being my hero, you are one of the most treasured gifts in my life.

My "Polarity Sister" Fran Burke, for sparking my research which led to this book.

Robert G Allen, my coach and mentor, for challenging me into writing this book. Thank you for sharing your wisdom and expertise so that I can become more of who I am meant to be.

Ann McIndoo, my author's coach, and her team – Mishael and Katie – for all your creative input and guidance in helping me see beyond the writing and the publication of this book.

To David Yoder and the Balboa Press team, for your assistance and patience, you made this experience enjoyable and easier.

Sher Smith, my Polarity Therapy and Brain Gym® instructor, and mentor, for providing such a great learning centre where everyone can "realize their potential". (www.realizingyourpotential.ca)

Dr. Karim Dhanani, my naturopathic doctor, Dr. Adam Chen, my TCM physician, and Jeanette Bakker, my Matrix Repatterning® practitioner, thank you for helping me remain balanced during this project.

The FIY Master Mind Team, (Heather, Colin, Larry, Peter, Roman, Anna, Nicky, Dinesh) for our weekly support calls, your assistance, and for cheering me on. When I am with you, I feel carried and uplifted to reach new heights. I look forward to reading your books!

Mes chers parents, Gaston et Ghislaine Bourgeois, en plus de la vie, je vous dois ma passion pour la lecture et la bonne bouffe. Votre amour, votre soutien et vos encouragements me permettent de me rendre jusqu'au bout de mes projets avec persévérance et fierté.

The Hoy family, for sharing the best of the Chinese culture with me, and for creating such a loving space within your family for me. Thank you, Baba Bing, Lily Ma, my "brothers" Edmond, Roland, Gordon, my "sisters" Shirley, Rita, and Bonnie, and their spouses, partners and children.

To my clients, for the pleasure and the privilege of working with you, for teaching me as much as I share with you.

And you, my readers, who are looking for answers to regain and maintain vibrant health; even though I haven't met you yet, I wish you the very best, especially a long, happy and vibrant life. I hope you will find this nourishment-for-wellness book to be useful, practical and life-transforming for you and your loved ones. Thank you for investing in this book and sharing it with others.

I welcome your comments, questions and feedback on my website at www.olivestolychees.com.

And finally, my deepest gratitude goes to my Divine Connections for their daily loving guidance, creative inspiration, and protection.

From the bottom of my heart,
Merci! Merci! Merci!
I LOVE you all!
Namasté!

This book is **Volume 1** of the *Olives to Lychees* collection focusing on nourishment for wellness. If you would like to experiment with more Everyday Mediter-asian Paleo spa recipes and learn about the Art of Feeling Well, the 5 elements and how to create your own calming spa environment at home, make sure you get your copy of **Volume 2** of *Olives to Lychees, Everyday Mediter-asian Spa Cuisine*.

A special offer:

If you enjoyed the Everyday Mediter-asian Paleo spa recipes in this book and would like to have more,
I invite you to create variations or new recipes along this theme, and share them with me at
www.olivestolychees.com. Send me your recipe and a brief explanation of what inspired you.
Make sure you include your name and email address.
If your recipe is chosen, it will be featured in a special chapter of my future book,
and you will receive a **free** copy of that book when it is printed.

Thank you for allowing me to be part of your life.

Merci beaucoup et bon appétit!

*May you be blessed
with an abundance of vibrant health, wealth, love, success and happiness
above and beyond what you could ask or imagine.
You deserve it all, and so does your family!*

Your friend, your witness, your cheerleader
Marie~Claire

Resources and Recommended Reading

Books

1. *The Matrix Repatterning Program for Pain Relief, Self-treatment for Musculoskeletal Pain* by George Roth, DC, ND (New Harbinger Publication Inc., 2005)
2. *Wheat Belly* by William Davis, MD (Rodale, 2011)
3. *Merriam-Webster's Collegiate Dictionary Eleventh Edition* (Springfield, Massachusetts, 2003)
4. *Wheat Belly Cookbook, 150 Recipes to Help You Lose the Wheat, Lose the Weight, and Find Your Path Back to Health* by William Davis, MD (Collins, 2013)
5. *Wheat Belly, 30-minute (or less!) Cookbook* by William Davis, MD (Collins, 2013)
6. *Fat Chance, Beating the Odds Against Sugar, Processed Food, Obesity, and Disease* by Robert H. Lustig, MD (Hudson Street Press, 2013)
7. *Salt Sugar Fat, How the Food Giants Hooked Us* by Michael Moss (Signal M&S, 2013)
8. *The Virgin Diet, Why Food Intolerance is the Real Cause of Weight Gain* by JJ Virgin (Harlequin, 2012)
9. *Food Rules, an eater's manual* by Michael Pollan (Penguin, 2009)
10. *In Defense of Food, an eater's manifesto* by Michael Pollan (Penguin, 2009)
11. *Cooked, a Natural History of Transformation* by Michael Pollan (The Penguin Press, 2013)
12. *Eat to Live, the Amazing Nutrient-rich Program for Fast and Sustained Weight Loss* by Joel Fuhrman, MD (Little, Brown and Company, 2012)
13. *French Women Don't Get Fat, the Secret of Eating for Pleasure* by Mireille Guiliano (Alfred A. Knopf, 2005)
14. *The End of Overeating, Taking Control of the Insatiable North American Appetite* by David A. Kessler, MD (McClelland & Stewart, 2010)
15. *The Acid-Alkaline Diet for Optimum Health, Restore your Health by Creating Balance in Your Diet,* Christopher Vasey, N.D. (Healing Arts Press, 2003)
16. *The Alkaline Cure, Lose Weight, Gain Energy and Feel Young,* Dr. Stephan Domenig (Harlequin, 2014)
17. *Mindless Eating, Why We Eat More Than We Think* by Brian Wansink, Ph.D. (Bantam Books, 2007)
18. *The Life Force Diet, 3 weeks to Supercharge your Health and Get Slim with Enzyme-rich Foods* by Michelle Schoffro Cook (Wiley, 2009)
19. *Mindful Eating, a Guide to Rediscovering a Healthy and Joyful Relationship with Food* by Jan Chozen Bays, MD (Shambhala, 2009)
20. *Clean up Your Diet, the Pure Food Program to Cleanse, Energize, and Revitalize* by Max Tomlinson (Duncan Baird Publishers, 2007)
21. *Intuitive Eating, a Revolutionary Program That Works* by Evelyn Tribole and Elyse Resch (St. Martin's Griffin, 2013)
22. *Food Matters, a Guide to Conscious Eating* by Mark Bittman (Simon & Schuster, 2009)
23. *Women, Food and God, an Unexpected Path to Almost Everything* by Geneen Roth (Scribner, 2010)
24. *Real Food, What to Eat and Why* by Nina Planck (Bloomsbury, 2006)
25. *Constant Craving, What Your Food Cravings Mean and How to Overcome Them* by Doreen Virtue (Hay House, 2011)
26. *Culinary Intelligence, the Art of Eating Healthy (and Really Well)* by Peter Kaminsky, (Vintage Books, 2013)
27. *What Are You Hungry For? The Chopra Solution to Permanent Weight Loss, Well-being, and Lightness of Soul* by Deepak Chopra (Crown Publishing Group, 2013)
28. *Food Energetics, the Spiritual, Emotional, and Nutritional Power of What We Eat* by Steve Gagné (Healing Arts Press, 2008)
29. *Against All Grains, Delectable Paleo Recipes to Eat Well & Feel Great* by Danielle Walker (Victory Belt Publishing Inc., 2013)
30. *Your Personal Paleo Code, the 3-step Plan to Lose Weight, Reverse Disease, and Stay Fit and Healthy for Life* by Chris Kresser, (Little, Brown and Company, 2013)
31. *The Polarity Process, Energy as a Healing Art* by Franklyn Sills (North Atlantic Books, 2001)
32. *Polarity Therapy Certification Training Manuals 1-3* by Sher Smith (2002)
33. *Radiant Body, Restful Mind, A Woman's Book of Comfort,* by Shubhra Krishan (New World Library, 2004)
34. *Quinta Essentia* by Morag Campbell (Masterworks, 1995)

Magazines

Paleo Magazine
Simply Guten Free

Index

The **bolded** text represents the recipe titles.

A

A Liquid Soup for Lunch 34
Alkaline morning tonic 33
Almond 15, 25, 28, 30, 35, 37, 40, 51–54, 72, 79–80, 85–87, 89–90, 92–95
Anchovies 40, 56–57, 61
Appetizers 25, 38, 40–43
Apples 28–30, 33–36, 38, 87, 95
Artichokes 58
Arugula 25, 52, 61
Asian Crackers 94
Asparagus 27, 43, 57

B

Bacon 41, 46, 69, 93
Bananapple Muffins with Spices 95
Basil 25–26, 34, 40–43, 50, 55–57, 60, 63–67, 73, 78–80, 83, 92
Bean sprouts 63, 70
Beet 34, 62
Blended beverages 33
Blue cheese 62, 85
Bocconcini 42
Bok choi 7, 70
Breakfast 6, 8, 14, 16, 24–26, 28–30, 35, 49, 51, 77, 81, 84, 93
Breakfast Almond Buns 93
Broccoli 7, 63–65, 70

C

Cantaloupe 7, 42, 85, 87
Cantaloupe and Figs with Honey and Blue Cheese 85
Capers 40, 57, 62, 64, 75
Carrot 7, 30, 34–35, 43, 46–56, 62, 64–66, 69, 72–74, 78
Carrot juice 34–35
Cashews 28, 30, 40, 55–56, 63
Cauliflower 43, 58–59, 62–65
Celery 30, 34, 39, 41, 45–50, 54, 66, 69, 73–74, 78
Cheese 4, 20, 23, 26, 42, 44, 58, 61–62, 83, 85

Chicken livers 38
Chicken stock 49–50, 69–70
Chicken Tagine with Olives and Preserved Lemons 67
Chinese Chicken Hot Pot 70
Chinese Wrapper-less Wonton Soup 47
Chorizo 42, 75
Coconut milk 15, 35, 44, 48, 79, 89
Complete Breakfast Smoothie 35
Coq au vin 23, 69
Crab 50
Cranshaw melon 45
Create-Your-Own Breakfast Cereal 28
Crème de citrouille 46
Crevettes et légumes avec leur sauce verte 43
Cucumber 7, 26, 31, 34, 39–40, 45, 53–54, 57, 60, 63, 73

D

Dark chocolate 6, 30, 36–37, 86
Desserts 6, 8, 14, 17, 25, 27, 29, 32, 46, 51, 81–87, 89–91, 93
Detox Blend 34
Dried apricots 85

E

Egg Crêpes 27, 29, 44, 49
Enoki mushrooms 45
Exotic Fruit Salad 25

F

Feta 42, 58, 61
Fish 3–4, 15–16, 45, 48, 50, 53, 56–57, 63, 70–71, 77–78
Fish or Seafood Stock 50
The Five 'C' Salad 55
Flavoured Whipped Cream 90
Fraises au poivre 84
French Chicken and Vegetable Galantine 41
French-style Scrambled Eggs 26

G

Gelatin 39–41, 49, 89–90
Grapes 7, 25, 42, 64, 84, 87–88
Grapes with Ginger, Lime and Mint 84
Greek Roasted Potatoes 60
Greek Shrimp Salad 57
Greek Souvlaki and Tzatziki 72
Greek Vegetable Kebabs 59
Greek Village Salad 60
Green beans 42, 61, 64, 79
Green Beans with Pancetta and Fried Shallots 61
Green Power Drink 34
Green tea 30–32, 34
Gremolata 73–74
Grilled Moroccan Lamb Skewers 74
Grilled Surf & Turf 75

H

Honeydew melon 45

I

I-have-a-cold-and-I-don't-feel-too-well Comfort Tea 33
Indian-spiced Fruit in an Almond Milk Bath 89
Italian Panna Cotta 89
Italian Stracciatella 44

J

Japanese Avocado and Wakame Salad 53
Japanese Lychees and Melon Salad 83

K

Kale 7, 34

L

Lamb 71–76
Leeks 7, 48, 50
Lemon Mint Ginger Tisane 33

Lobster 50
Lover's tea blend 32
Lychees 25, 42, 71, 83, 87–89, 97

M

Macadamia v, 4, 28, 35, 40
Make-Me-Feel-Better Drink 34
Manchego 42
Mandarin Orange Almond Salad 54
Mandarin oranges 54, 87
Mango 7, 25, 28, 30, 35, 42, 45, 55–56, 87–89
Mascarpone cheese 83
Matcha 31–32, 34
Mediter-asian Cocktail Skewers 42
Mediterranean Date and Orange Salad 85
Mediterranean Herb Loaf 92
Medjool dates 53, 90
Melon 31, 42, 45, 83
Moroccan Chicken Stew 68
Moroccan Mint Tea 32
Moroccan Roasted Red Peppers Salad 52
Moroccan Tagine of Lamb, Vegetables and Prunes 71
Mousse au saumon 39
Mozzarella 42, 73–74
Mushrooms 27, 41, 45, 47, 50, 59, 69–70

N

Nectarines 27, 82, 87
No-fuss Baked Chicken Dinner 66

O

Orange 7, 29–31, 33–36, 43, 45, 52–55, 57–58, 61, 63–64, 66, 72–75, 79–81, 84–88, 91
Orange and Carrot Salad with Pancetta Crisps 52
Orange blossom water 53
Orange marmalade 52
Osso Buco alla Milanese 73

P

Pancetta 38–39, 41, 52–53, 61, 69
Papaya 7, 35, 45, 88–89
Parmesan 25–26, 48, 52, 93
Parsnips 49–50, 72
Pâté de foies de poulet 38
Peaches 7, 27, 31, 82, 87
Peaches Cardinal 82
Pears 28, 87, 95
Peas 7, 42, 57, 63, 79, 93
Pecans 30, 40
Pep-To-Cu 34
Pesto 42
Pineapple 25, 27, 42, 81–82, 87–89
Pineapple with Mint Paste 82
Poached Peaches 87
Pomegranate 25, 82–83, 86, 89
Potatoes 2, 7, 27, 43, 48, 57, 60, 62, 68, 71–74, 79
Preserved lemons 52, 67–68
Prosciutto 42, 62
Prunes 71–72
Pumpkin 28, 30, 46

Q

Quick and Portable Breakfast Ideas 25

R

Raisins 62, 92–93, 95
Raspberries 82, 86
Red Grapefruit and Pomegranate Salad 86
Roasted Grapes with Mascarpone Cream 88
Roasted Sicilian Cauliflower 62
Rose water 86

S

Salade de légumes marinés 64
Salade niçoise 56
Salami 42
Sambal Oelek 56, 63, 70
Sardinian Cauliflower 58
Satisfying Trail Mix 30
Sautéed Scallops with Piment d'Espelette and Lime 77
Seaweed 53
Semisweet chocolate 86
Shredded Carrots with Toasted Almonds 51
Shrimp 16, 27, 42–43, 45, 47–48, 50, 53–58, 63, 70, 75–76, 79–80
Simple Chicken Soup 49
Smoked salmon 40, 64
Smoothies 20, 30–31, 33–35
Snacks 8, 15–16, 18, 25, 29–30, 35, 38, 40, 44, 94
Snow peas 42, 57, 63
Soups 16, 20, 25, 27, 34, 43–50, 62, 66, 70, 74
Spanish Gazpacho 45
Spanish Hot Chocolate 36
Spanish-inspired "Chocolado" Pudding-like Mousse 90
Spanish Shrimp and Tomatoes 79
Spanish Tortilla 27
Spiced Apple Cider 36
Spiced Applesauce 29
Spiced Nuts 40
Spinach 7, 34–35, 43, 45, 56, 59, 64, 79
Spinach Salad with Red Grapes and Smoked Salmon Roses 64
Steamed Vegetables with Tomato Dressing 63
Stews 16, 47, 67–69, 71, 79
Strawberries with Balsamic Vinegar 83
Sugar snaps 57
Sun-dried tomatoes 40–41, 66, 93
Sun-dried Tomato Tapenade 40

T

Tahini 54
Tapas 17, 38
Thai Beef Salad 63
Thai Butternut Squash and Shrimp Curry 47
Thai Curried Shrimp 79
Thai Green Mango Salad 55
Thai Scallops and Spinach Soup 45
Thai Steamed Fish 78
Thai Tropical Fruit Salad with a Papaya Sauce 88
Tisanes 31, 33
Tomatoes 7, 15, 18, 25, 30, 34, 40–43, 45, 50, 53–54, 57, 59–60, 63–66, 70, 73–75, 79–80, 93
Trois fondues au chocolat 86
Tropical Green Shake 35
Turkey 41, 47, 66
Turmeric 34, 48, 68, 71

U

Unsweetened cocoa 37, 91

V

Veal 47, 73
Vegetables Dishes 8, 51, 67, 72
Vegetable Stock 50
Vichyssoise 48

W

Walnuts 28, 30, 35, 40, 93
Water chestnuts 47
Watermelon 7, 42, 83
White chocolate 87
White miso 54
Wilted Spinach with Fried Garlic 59

Y

Yellow beans 43
Yogurt 4, 23, 29, 39, 73, 91

Z

Zucchini 7, 43, 50, 59, 62, 70, 72, 75, 79

CPSIA information can be obtained at www.ICGtesting.com
Printed in the USA
LVOW05s1918170315

430865LV00003B/7/P